Child and Adolescent
Psychopharmacology

DEVELOPMENTAL CLINICAL PSYCHOLOGY AND PSYCHIATRY SERIES

Series Editor: **Alan E. Kazdin**

In the Series:

Child and Adolescent Psychopharmacology

Magda Campbell
Wayne H. Green
Stephen I. Deutsch

Volume 2.
Developmental Clinical Psychology and Psychiatry

 SAGE Publications   Beverly Hills   London   New Delhi

For information address:

SAGE Publications, Inc.
275 South Beverly Drive
Beverly Hills, California 90212

SAGE Publications India Pvt. Ltd.
M-32 Market
Greater Kailash I
New Delhi 110 048 India

SAGE Publications Ltd
28 Banner Street
London EC1Y 8QE
England

Printed in the United States of America

Library of Congress Cataloging in Publication Data

Campbell, Magda.
    Child and adolescent psychopharmacology.

    (Developmental clinical psychology and psychiatry ; v. 2)
    Bibliography: p.
    Includes index.
    1. Pediatric psychopharmacology. 2. Psychotropic
drugs. I. Green, Wayne H. II. Deutsch, Stephen I.
III. Title. IV. Series. [DNLM: 1. Drug Therapy—in
infancy and childhood. W1 DE997NC v. 2 / WS 366 C189c]
RJ504.7.C36 1985   615'.78   85-2190
ISBN 0-8039-2463-1
ISBN 0-8039-2464-X (pbk.)

FIRST PRINTING

CONTENTS

SERIES EDITOR'S INTRODUCTION

Interest in child development and adjustment is by no means new. Yet, only recently has the study of children benefitted from advances in both clinical and scientific research. Many reasons might explain the recent systematic attention to children, including more pervasive advances in research in the social and biological sciences, the emergence of disciplines and subdisciplines that focus exclusively on childhood and adolescence, and greater appreciation of the impact of such influences as the family, peers, school, and many other factors on child adjustment. Apart from interest in the study of child development and adjustment for its own sake, the need to address clinical problems of adulthood naturally draws one to investigation of precursors in childhood and adolescence.

Within a relatively brief period, the study of childhood development, child psychopathology, and child mental health has evolved and proliferated considerably. In fact, several different professional journals, annual book series, and handbooks devoted entirely to the study of children and adolescents and their adjustment document the proliferation of work in the field. Although many different disciplines and specialty areas contribute to knowledge of childhood disorders, there is a paucity of resource materials that present information in an authoritative, systematic, and disseminable fashion. There is a need within the field to present latest developments and to represent different disciplines and conceptual views of and multiple approaches to the topics of childhood adjustment and maladjustment.

The Sage Series in Developmental Clinical Psychology and Psychiatry is designed to serve uniquely several needs of the field. The series encompasses individual monographs prepared by experts in the fields of clinical child psychology, child psychiatry, child development, and related disciplines. The primary focus is on childhood psychopathology, which refers broadly here to the diagnosis, assessment, treatment, and prevention of problems of children and adolescents. The scope of the series is necessarily broad because of the working assumption—if not demonstrated fact—that understanding, identifying, and treating problems of youth regrettably cannot be resolved by narrow, single discipline, and parochial conceptual views. Commitment to the goal of understanding childhood disorders requires the sacrifice of professional parochialism. Thus, the series draws upon multiple disciplines and diverse views within a given discipline.

The task for individual contributors is to present the latest theory and research on various topics including specific types of dysfunction, diagnostic and treatment approaches, and special problem areas that affect adjustment. Core topics within child clinical work are addressed by the series. Authors are asked to bridge potential theory and research, research and clinical practice, and current status and future directions. The goals of the series and the tasks presented to individual contributors are demanding. We have been extremely fortunate in recruiting leaders in the fields who have been able to translate their recognized scholarship and expertise into highly readable works on contemporary topics.

The present monograph has been prepared by Drs. Magda Campbell, Wayne H. Green, and Stephen I. Deutsch on the topic of childhood pharmacotherapy. The topic is of obvious significance given the advances both in research and clinical uses of medication with children. This monograph is unique in conveying both the substantive findings and methodological issues of the field. Issues regarding the design of medication trials and measurement of the efficacy and safety of pharmacological treatments are fully elaborated. Individual classes of medication are carefully reviewed. The findings are thoroughly presented and incisively evaluated in a way that reflects a rare combination of scholarship and clinical usefulness. The book is an authoritative treatise without peer, in part because it was prepared by a group whose contributions to the topic have already been so influential.

Alan E. Kazdin, Ph.D.

PREFACE

Pharmacotherapy is an important and at times essential intervention in the comprehensive and highly individualized treatment plan, developed to meet the needs of the moderately to severely disturbed child or adolescent. This book was designed to present mental health professionals with the current status of pharmacotherapy of psychiatric disorders occurring in this young age group. Physicians will find a practical guide to dosage, indications, and side effects. The book will be of particular interest to advanced undergraduate and graduate students in psychology, and medical students and house officers in pediatrics and psychiatry. The reader will find it a valuable source of primary references.

This book was not intended to be an exhaustive, detailed review of all pharmacological studies in children; the constraints imposed by the page limitation would make this an impossible task. Rather, we chose to selectively and critically review the seminal studies and provide a flavor of the historical developments in this burgeoning field. Most of the investigations covered in this book were conducted in a placebo-controlled, double-blind manner with a cohort of patients identified according to operational diagnostic criteria.

There is a deliberate imbalance to the emphasis of our presentation; specifically, in the Assessments section, emphasis was placed on measures and issues relating to untoward effects. This section presents an overview of the techniques and methods currently available to assess the untoward effects of psychoactive drugs. These tools are essential in developing a more scientific and safe use of drugs in the treatment of psychiatric patients. They are of use to the researcher in determining the risk-benefit ratio of old and new drugs, to the clinician in following an individual patient's progress on a given drug, and in comparing drugs. It is essential that new and increasingly refined assessment techniques for side effects and more rigorous documentation accompany the current trends in psychiatry toward greater refinement of diagnosis and pharmacologic specificity. The majority of these measures were developed for adult patients—the same population from which most of our current information regarding short- and long-term toxicity is derived. Unfortunately, this important area has been neglected in childhood and adolescence (Shader & DiMascio, 1970). Also, in our consideration of the specific classes of drugs, a subsection of each chapter is devoted to a discussion of immediate and long-term untoward effects. It is our feeling that prior to prescribing a drug to a developing child, a critical assessment of the risk-benefit ratio for the given child must be made. Drugs should be reserved only for definite indications and when the severity of symptoms interferes with development and learning.

A detailed discussion of issues pertaining to bioavailability, pharmacokinetics, and the utility of plasma levels for most drugs was omitted. A comprehensive and recent review of drug levels in blood in childhood psychopharmacology is available (Gualtieri, Golden, et al., 1984). The section on tricyclic antidepressants is an exception; in this chapter, the important role of plasma levels in ensuring antidepressant efficacy and minimizing toxicity is considered in some depth. Issues pertaining to chemical structure of psychoactive drugs and their metabolism were beyond the scope of our considerations: These areas have been amply covered in a comprehensive textbook by Klein et al. (1980).

After concluding our review of the major drug classes and their indications, we remain impressed by the growth of the field in the past five years and the urgent need for continued research. The prognosis for many of the psychiatric disorders in childhood is at best guarded (Robins, 1966), and remains so despite a variety of available interventions today, including pharmacotherapy. Further drug research should provide more effective and safer interventions. Moreover, studies should be designed to measure the comparative efficacy of psychosocial and pharmacological interventions, as well as their interaction. We would be gratified if our book would stimulate further studies in these areas. This work was supported in part by NIMH grants MH-32212 and MH-40177 to Dr. Campbell.

1

INTRODUCTION

CLINICAL TRIALS AND EXPERIMENTAL DESIGN

When the investigator wishes to assess the safety, efficacy, and indications of a new psychoactive agent a systematic series of experiments is undertaken (for review, see General Considerations for the Clinical Evaluation of Drugs, 1977; Guidelines for the Clinical Evaluation of Psychoactive Drugs in Infants and Children, 1979; Sprague, 1978). The researcher usually starts with a single or time-limited multiple dose open trial, progresses to a single-blind study, and finally to a double-blind and controlled study with an adequate sample size. Only when the efficacy and long-term safety of a drug have been established should the practitioner prescribe the medication.

Though carefully conducted uncontrolled trials have brought valuable information (e.g., Bradley's (1937) study of amphetamine; Weinberg et al.'s (1973) study of an antidepressant), controlled trials are required for the critical assessment of efficacy. Drug-induced changes in patients are seldom dramatic, and because the physician, parent, and child may have preconceived expectations from the treatment, double-blind studies are essential. Furthermore, spontaneous improvement may occur, or admission to the hospital and placement in a structured therapeutic milieu itself may decrease the symptoms (Campbell, Small et al., 1984). Even when effective drugs are employed, about 30 percent of patients improve with placebo. All of these variables can be controlled by employing double-blind and placebo-controlled procedures.

A clinical trial of a new drug requires careful planning. First the questions that one wishes to answer should be specified. The questions should be few in number and precise. It should be specified how these aims are to be achieved and what methods will be used. Basic decisions must be made before attempting to fit the experimental question into a research design. The decision should be made as to whether the new treatment should be compared to a placebo, to a standard drug, or whether two treatments are to be compared against each other with a placebo used for a control. If a trial has more than two treatment groups, careful designs are required, and the issues of carryover (lasting effects of therapy) and drug washout must be taken into consideration (Chassan, 1979; Cochran & Cox, 1957; Laska et al., 1983).

Early planning stages must include a detailed description of patients to be studied. These include the diagnosis, inclusion and exclusion criteria, and a variety of demographic information. In children, the sample should be as homogeneous as possible in respect to chronological age. Patient selection is very important. The sample has to be representative and the sample size adequate. The outcome may be affected by such variables as symptom severity, inpatient or outpatient status, IQ, or chronicity of illness.

In order to reduce bias, patients should be randomly assigned to treatments. Stratified random assignments may be used if a certain patient characteristic, such as IQ or age, will influence treatment outcome. Matching is an unresolved problem in pediatric psychopharmacology, because it is not known which variables should be matched (Fish, 1968). In addition, matching is difficult for practical reasons because patients are usually admitted over a period of time, and it is never known if a better match will come along later.

Baseline considerations are crucial to the proper design of the study. Since the symptoms in children are known to fluctuate from setting to setting (Conners, 1985), a stable baseline is needed before commencing drug treatment. This can usually be established in two weeks and should include at least two ratings while the subject receives placebo.

A baseline placebo period serves more than one function: It ensures washout, it helps the child to get used to taking the medication, and it identifies placebo responders. Placebo responders exist even among severely disturbed patients whose lack of response to outpatient treatment led to hospitalization. For example, of 82 such children diagnosed as conduct disorder, undersocialized, aggressive type, with a behavioral profile of severe explosiveness and disruptiveness, 16 were dropped from a double-blind and placebo-controlled clinical trial during the 2-week baseline placebo period because severe aggressiveness and explosiveness ceased by the end of the 2-week baseline period (Campbell, Small, et al., 1984).

A sine qua non of a successful drug trial is compliance, that is, the patient actually consuming the medication. A common cause for failure to respond to pharmacotherapy is noncompliance, but little attention has been paid to this issue in pediatric psychopharmacology. Treatment compliance in adult psychiatric patients was carefully reviewed by Blackwell (1982).

For general discussion, experimental designs can be divided into two major categories; extensive (between group) and intensive (within individual) designs.

In the *extensive design* the medication under study is analyzed across groups of patients. For example, the most common design would randomly assign one group of patients to an active medication and contrast its effects to a group that receives a placebo *(comparative or parallel design)*. The percentage of patients who improve in the medication group is compared with the percentage who improve in the placebo group. Examples of extensive designs are the crossover study in which the percentage of patients who improve after switching from medication to placebo is compared to the percentage who improve after changing from placebo to medication; the sequential design, in which sample size is determined by statistical procedures following each observation; and the factorial design, which is useful in increasing statistical power and minimizing bias due to uneven distribution of patient characteristics between treatment groups. An important point about all extensive designs is that the percentage change (or mean change) always pertains to groups of patients.

In the intensive design the effect of the investigational medication is studied within individual patients. The most common procedure would be to alternate between medication and placebo periods in a single patient. With intensive designs, changes in a patient's behavior during a waiting period or placebo period are compared with changes in that same patient after treatment. This design is particularly useful in assessing treatment effects in rare conditions because it circumvents the problem of obtaining an equivalent sample of patients for a control group. The essence of the intensive design is that it allows testing for true differential treatment effects in relation to the individual patient; thus, the investigator is not restricted to group statistics when assessing drug efficacy. The intensive design also allows some estimate of trend effects within the patient.

A major problem with the intensive design is that it requires the behavior in question to be relatively stable over time. Thus, information must be available on the natural history of the disease. The investigator must be confident that the behavior is stable during the premedication phase (baseline period) and demonstrate that it changes abruptly when treatment is introduced. A practical difficulty is that intensive designs require a longer time commitment than extensive designs. If the patient is only available for a short period, intensive designs are usually ruled out. Another problem is that intensive designs cannot be used when the medication being tested has long-lasting carry-over effects. If the effect of the medication is irreversible, the design cannot be used. If the carry-over effect is brief, the researcher must know its duration and allow for ample "washout." Experimental designs and various methodological issues are discussed in detail by Chassan (1979), Bradford Hill (1971), Kazdin (1981), Conners (1977), and Sprague (1978).

ASSESSMENT

Rating Conditions

Behavioral and other drug-dependent variables should be assessed at fixed points, not long after drug ingestion, preferably in the morning. Rating conditions (e.g., classroom, playroom, office, familiar or unfamiliar environment, standard fixed stimulus environment) may markedly influence response to drug, or neuroleptic-related dyskinesias. Gleser (1968) discussed issues concerning rating conditions.

Efficacy

The ability to measure the therapeutic efficacy of a psychoactive agent will not only depend on the patient's response, but also on the sensitivity of the measuring instrument to change due to drug. In growing organisms, such as children, developmental factors must be taken into account (Conners, 1985; Hardesty, 1982). Pediatric psychopharmacology is troubled by problems of measurement (Campbell, 1979; Conners, 1985; Fish, 1968; Hardesty, 1982; Werry, 1978). This section will summarize the highlights of treatment assessment.

Instruments measuring abnormal behavior can be classified into a variety of categories, depending on what they measure, how they measure it, and who is doing the measurement. With regard to what is being measured, instruments assessing abnormal behavior (or psychopathology) can be classified into three major categories. The first category is composed of instruments developed for purposes of diagnosis: for example, the NIMH Diagnostic Interview Schedule for Children (DISC, based on a scale developed by Herjanic & Campbell, 1977); Kiddie-SADS (K-SADS, in Chambers et al., 1978); Bellevue Index of Depression (BID, in Petti, 1978); Children's Depression Rating Scale (CDRS, see Poznanski et al., 1979). The second category is composed of scales assessing behavioral profiles in a variety of clinical diagnostic groups: for example, Children's Psychiatric Rating Scale (CPRS, *Psychopharmacology Bulletin,* 1973); Children's Behavior Inventory (CBI, see Burdock & Hardesty, 1967); Child Behavior Checklist (CBCL, in Achenbach, 1978; Achenbach & Edelbrock, 1979); Conners' Parent Questionnaire (CPQ), Conners' Teacher Questionnaire (CTQ), Conners' Parent-Teacher Questionnaire (PTQ, *Psychopharmacology Bulletin,* 1973). In the third category are scales sensitive enough to reflect treatment-related changes. Most of these scales come from the two previous categories: for example, all three Conners scales, CPRS, and the K-SADS. The Clinical Global Impressions (CGI, in *Psychopharmacology Bulletin,* 1973), is widely used and sensitive to drug-induced changes.

For the measurement of psychopathology, the instruments can be divided into three categories: objective behavior observation, subjective rating scales, and mechanical devices. Objective observation tools usually record the frequencies of select behaviors over fixed periods of time. This can be accomplished by direct sampling methods with fixed periods of observation. For example, the Timed Stereotypies Rating Scale is currently being used in studies of haloperidol in autistic children (Perry et al., 1985). Objective Rating Scales were reviewed by Werry (1979) and Conners (1985). Although the direct time sampling method is accurate, the most important criticisms of objective rating scales are that they are not necessarily sensitive to change due to drug, and worse, that they may not be valid indications of improvement (Conners, 1985). Also, the presence of an observer may change the very behavior—such as aggressiveness and explosiveness—for which the drug has been prescribed (Campbell, Small, et al., 1984). Finally, this method is time-consuming and requires highly trained observers.

Mechanical or electronic devices are occasionally used. Campbell, Anderson, Small, et al. (1982) and Anderson et al. (1984) used pressure sensors mounted under carpeting and connected with a computer to measure hyperactivity and general motor activity in young autistic children, as well as the duration of stereotypies. Rapoport, Buchsbaum et al. (1978) used an actometer attached to the wrist or waistline of hyperactive children to measure the hyperactivity and its changes when they were awake and asleep. For review, Werry (1979) is recommended. Video tapes may be useful. Videotaping of patient's examination, interview or free-play, can be subsequently rated by independent raters who are blind to the study design and/or patient's identity. These videotaped samples should not be presented in chronological order, but rather randomized. The method has been used in assessing haloperidal treatment effects (Campbell, Anderson, et al., 1978; Campbell, in preparation) and drug safety (tardive and withdrawal dyskinesias) in autistic children (Perry et al., 1985). In the case of neuroleptic-related dyskinesias, live ratings were very close to ratngs of videotapes (Perry et al., 1985).

The most commonly employed method in children's psychopharmacology is the use of rating scales. These are subjective instruments, usually measuring the severity of symptoms on a scale (e.g., the CPRS), or categorical, recording the presence or the absence of a behavior (e.g., CBI). The latter type is usually not sensitive to change due to drug, because often a symptom (or symptoms) is not entirely eliminated by administration of a drug over a period of a few weeks, as in most clinical trials (Campbell, Anderson, et al., 1978; Conners, 1985). Scales can be multi-item (e.g., CPRS, CBI) or global, such as the CGI. Usually a global scale is more sensitive and more efficient.

With respect to who is doing the measurement, the scales can be divided into the following categories: physician (e.g., CPRS, CGI, K-SADS), nurse (e.g., CTQ, PTQ) parent (e.g., CPQ, PTQ), and self-report or self-rating scales (e.g., Children's Depression Inventory, CDI, Kovacs, 1980/81; Short Children's Depression Inventory, SCDI, Carlson & Cantwell, 1979; Profile of Mood States, POMS, adapted for children by Walker, 1982).

Most scales specify the appropriate chronological age range and were developed for children ages 6 to 12. However, some of these scales are also appropriate for younger adolescents (e.g., K-SADS, CBI). Scales appropriate for younger children are the PTQ and the first 28 items of CPRS (mainly for autistics).

In adolescents the Brief Psychiatric Rating Scale (BPRS) developed by Overall and Gorham (1962), and the CGI have been used (Pool et al., 1976; Realmuto et al., 1984). The BPRS was developed for evaluation of change in adult patients and was intended to be used by professionals, mainly physicians. Both studies of adolescents involved schizophrenics. Because drug effects were significant, it seems appropriate to use adult scales for adolescent schizophrenics.

The most widely used and researched rating scales are those of Conners. The PTQ, CPQ, and CTQ are appropriate for hyperactive and conduct disorder children. The 10-item PTQ, an abridged form, is a very sensitive instrument for measuring drug-induced change in a variety of psychiatric disorders of children. The CPRS was developed by the Psychopharmacology Research Branch of the NIMH (*Psychopharmacology Bulletin,* 1973). It is composed of 63 behavioral items, rated on a scale ranging from 0 to 7. The first 28 items are based exclusively on observation; they are based on a scale developed by Fish (1968), and are appropriate for use with young autistic and retarded children. The subsequent items rely on the child's verbalization. The CPRS was used extensively in infantile autism (Anderson et al., 1984; Campbell, Anderson, Meier et al., 1978; Campbell, Anderson, Small et al., 1982; Campbell, Small et al., 1978) and in conduct disorder (Campbell, Cohen et al., 1982; Campbell, Small et al., 1984).

For an extensive review and analysis of children's behavioral instruments, with data on reliability, validity, and sensitivity, chapters by Werry (1978) and Conners (1985) are recommended, as are articles on depression scales by Kazdin (1981), Kazdin and Petti (1982), and Kazdin et al. (1983); and a special issue of the *Psychopharmacology Bulletin* (1973) on pharmacotherapy in children. In the near future, a revised and updated issue of *Psychopharmacology Bulletin* will be printed that should be the most comprehensive and informative document regarding assessment techniques for this age group of patients. (The Psychopharmacological, Biological and Physical Treatments Subcommittee of the NIMH will be responsible for this document.)

Safety (Measurement of Untoward Effects)

This section presents an overview of the techniques and methods currently available to assess the side effects of psychoactive medication. These tools are essential in developing a more scientific and safer use of psychoactive drugs in the treatment of psychiatric patients. They are of use to the researcher in determining the risk-benefit ratio of old and new drugs and to the clinician in following an individual patient's progress on a given drug and in comparing drugs. It is essential that new and increasingly refined assessment techniques for side effects and more rigorous documentation accompany the current trends in psychiatry toward greater refinement of diagnosis and pharmacologic specificity.

The physician should be acquainted with the untoward effects (or side effects) of the psychoactive drug he or she wishes to prescribe to the patient as much as with the therapeutic effects, and should share knowledge with the patient, and the patient's family. The doctor should acquire some baseline information on the systems he or she expects may be adversely affected by the drug in question: This may include a detailed history, laboratory data, electrocardiogram (EKG), kidney function, and a physical examination (e.g., for goiter). Each patient should be carefully monitored for possible untoward effects. Unnecessary dose escalations and polypharmacy should be avoided.

Our knowledge of side effects is best acquired from controlled trials before a drug is put on the market, and by continuing systematic observation and evaluation even after FDA approval has been granted. Controlled trials require large sample sizes, and they should be conducted under double-blind, placebo-controlled conditions. Such studies depend upon accurate and stable base rates for both side effects and for general behavior. Also, side effects must be rigorously defined and subject to reliable assessment (Klein et al., 1980). Such systematic research into side effects is scant at best.

This section will discuss the following topics:

(1) The available assessment methods for side effects:

checklists,

scales,

laboratory monitoring,

physical examination, and

neurogical examination.

(2) The side effects to be assessed:

behavioral toxicity: psychomotor and cognitive; personality and gross behavior, including mood states;

behavioral and other withdrawal effects;

central nervous system side effects: extrapyramidal side effects (i.e., acute dystonic reactions, dyskinesias, parkinsonian reactions, akathisia, rabbit syndrome); other central nervous system side effects; tardive and withdrawal dyskinesias;

supersensitivity psychosis;

electrophysiological side effects;

autonomic nervous system side effects;

cardiovascular side effects;

abnormal laboratory findings;

endocrine and metabolic side effects;

adverse effects of psychoactive drugs on IQ; and

adverse effects of psychoactive drugs on linear growth.

The purpose of this section is to give an overview of rating scales and other available assessment methods for documenting baseline measurements and adverse changes due to drug treatment. Such information is not only essential in the evaluation of new drugs, but is also helpful in routine clinical practice. Much of the current information is derived from adult data, and many of the instruments were developed for adults and are not necessarily appropriate for children. The section is organized by specific side effects. The currently available measures are highlighted and the most relevant literature reviews are given.

The rationale for the development of behavioral and neurological assessment measures and related psychometric issues will not be discussed here; for a comprehensive recent review of these subjects the following readings are recommended: Burdock (1982), Englesmann (1982), Guy (1982), Hamilton (1982), Simpson (1982), and Garfield (1982).

Assessment of ophthalmologic, dermatologic, allergic, and some other side effects (e.g., seizures) will not be discussed here, though they require recognition, examination, and appropriate medical attention. Concerning measures and methods in ophthalmology, a series of articles edited by Ederer (1975) is recommended.

Behavioral Toxicity

Behavioral toxicity means the deleterious alteration of behavior of a patient by a psychoactive agent (Holliday, 1967). DiMascio and Shader (1970, p. 127) give the following definition for behavioral toxicity: "Behavioral toxicity is a phrase used to denote those pharmacological actions of a drug that, when administered within the dosage range in which it has been found to possess clinical utility, produce—through mechanisms not immediately specifiable—alterations in perceptual and cognitive functions, psychomotor performance, motivation, mood, interpersonal relationships, or intrapsychic processes of an individual to the degree that they interfere with or limit the capacity of the individual to function within his setting or constitute a hazard to his physical well-being."

Thompson and Schuster (1968, p. 215) observe that all drugs can have adverse effects if administered at a wrong dosage, or under wrong conditions: "More specifically, behavioral toxicity must be defined in terms of the prevailing environmental conditions. If behavioral changes associated with drug administration are inappropriate under the existing environmental conditions (i.e., as compared with baseline behavior in the absence of the drug), the drug effects are behaviorally toxic. A given drug may be therapeutic for one organism under a given set of conditions but toxic to another organism under other conditions." For instance, lithium carbonate has a calming effect on the mood of patients with mania; when given to normal subjects it yields generalized subjective dysphoria (Judd, 1979). Thompson and Schuster (1968) list the following as examples of behaviorally toxic effects: atropine psychosis; impaired ability to concentrate due to diphenylhydantoin; agitation; anxiety, confusion, dizziness, drowsiness, euphoria, irritability, light-headedness, restlessness, tiredness, and weakness, resulting from a variety of psychoactive drugs. They emphasize that, "It should be obvious that the study of behavioral toxicity of drugs is simply an extension of the procedures used for the screening of the new compounds. Both functions may be served by the same procedures, and in this manner it is possible to assess not only a new compound's therapeutic efficacy but its potential behavioral toxicity as well" (Thompson & Schuster, 1968, p. 217). "By carefully selecting behavioral procedures for analysis . . . the investigator may be able to detect toxicity that would otherwise remain undetected" (Thompson & Schuster, 1968, p. 216).

Psychomotor and cognitive. Psychomotor functions are behaviors involving muscular activities in response to various environmental stimuli. Laboratory tests, such as reaction time and various performance tasks, have been developed to measure such functions. These laboratory tasks are related to, or may represent, elements of real-life tasks such as operating machines and motor vehicles.

Numerous laboratory tests are available to assess such cognitive functions as attention, memory, learning, retention, and others. The laboratory tests developed for the assessment of psychomotor and cognitive functions are the most objective measures in use in psychopharmacology; they are usually standardized. The effect of psychoactive drugs on psychomotor and cognitive functions may or may not be the same in normal individuals as in psychiatric patients. The effects may also be dose dependent.

Among all populations, perhaps the possible adverse effects of psychoactive drugs on cognition and learning in the mentally retarded are of greatest import. First, these individuals are of subnormal intelligence with severe learning problems; second, once they are placed on a neuroleptic drug, its administration is usually prolonged over many years. For a review of the pertinent literature in the mentally retarded, two chapters by Aman (1978, 1984) are recommended.

DiMascio and Shader (1970) reviewed the literature concerning the effects of neuroleptics, antidepressants, and antianxiety agents on psychomotor and cognitive functions; a more recent review is that of Wittenborn (1978). McNair (1973) presented a critical review of the effects of antianxiety drugs. The literature on children has been reviewed by Aman (1978), Campbell, Green et al. (1983) and Platt et al. (1984). Sprague (1973) is also recommended. Most of the reports indicate that these classes of drugs have adverse effects on psychomotor and cognitive functions as assessed by psychological laboratory tests. For example, in adult epileptic patients of normal intelligence, phenobarbital adversely affected speed of access to information in short-term memory, and it was highly sensitive to increased levels of the drug. At the two blood levels most commonly prescribed in epilepsy, speed of access to long-term memory was not similarly affected (MacLeod et al., 1978).

More recently, the effects of lithium carbonate on cognition, sensorymotor performance, and creativity using a variety of laboratory measures in normal subjects or patients have been reported (Judd, 1979; Judd, Hubbard, Janowsky, Huey & Takahashi, 1977; Linnoila et al., 1974; Platt et al., 1984; Schou, 1968, 1981; Small et al., 1972).

Personality and gross behavior including mood states. Judd (1979) and Judd, Hubbard, Janowsky, Huey, & Attewell (1977) have studied systematically the effect of lithium on personality in normals, using the California Psychological Inventory (Gough, 1969) and the Holtzman Ink Blot Technique (Holtzman, 1958); the differences, if any, between drug and placebo conditions were minimal. Gardos et al. (1968) have shown that benzodiazepines, particularly chlordiazepoxide, produce increased hostility and aggressiveness in volunteers as measured by the

Buss-Durkee Hostility Inventory (Buss & Durkee, 1957), and the Gottschalk-Gleser Hostility Scales (Gottschalk et al., 1963).

DiMascio et al. (1970, p. 134) discuss the untoward effects of psychoactive drugs on mood under two headings: paradoxical effects in a "direction opposite to the clinically desirable one for which the drug has been prescribed"—such as increased anxiety with benzodiazepines or worsening of depressive affect with imipramine; and pendular (effects in a direction that is desired but to a degree that the resulting mood state will be the opposite of the one for which the drug was initially prescribed)—such as chlorpromazine yielding depressive affect in manic patients.

Almost any behavior can be changed adversely by the administration of a psychoactive agent; this includes worsening of pre-existing symptoms, onset of acute psychotic symptoms in previously nonpsychotic individuals, and catatonic-like state, to name a few. In our twenty years of clinical and research experience with children, particularly of preschool age, behavioral toxicity is often seen long before any extrapyramidal, autonomic, or other untoward effects appear (Campbell, Anderson et al., 1982; Campbell, Green et al., 1983; Petti et al., 1982).

Findings of the effects of lithium on affect, mood, and behavior in normal volunteers have been reported by several authors. Some of the reports are anecdoctal, others employed self-rating scales, mood scales, rater observation, and adverse symptom checklists. Schou (1967, 1968) reported tiredness and muscular heaviness, emotional lability, inertia, increased irritability, and so on, depending on the dose administered. Small et al. (1972) reported reduction in alertness, mental clarity, efficiency, and impairment in work and school performance. Judd (1979) and Judd, Hubbard, Janowsky, Huey, and Takahashi (1977) used a variety of measures in their volunteers; in general, the ratings indicate that lithium at serum levels ranging from 0.7 to 1.4 mEq/q has adverse effects in the normals on mood and on other behaviors as measured by self-report scales (POMS, the Subjective State Questionnaire, and the Subjective High Assessment Scale), the Behavioral Observation Scale, and the "Significant Other" Questionnaire. It is of interest that the two independent raters who used the objective rating scale were not able to observe any differences in mood and behavior in the subjects on or off lithium maintenance, whereas the persons who knew the subjects more intimately and were close to them rated statistically significant worsening on lithium. This included drowsiness, diminished ability to work hard, and diminished ability to think clearly.

DiMascio and colleagues (DiMascio, Shader, & Giller, 1970; DiMascio, Shader, & Harmatz, 1970) and Klein et al. (1980) reviewed the pertinent literature involving the neuroleptics, antidepressants, and antianxiety agents.

The work of Rapoport, Buchsbaum et al. (1980) is most relevant concerning the adverse effects of dextroamphetamine on the mood of normal and attention deficit children (with hyperactivity) and its measurement.

Behavioral and Other Withdrawal Effects

As early as the sixties, but particularly in most recent years, increasing attention has been paid to the emergence of various symptoms and signs subsequent to the discontinuation of psychoactive drugs. These include worsening of pre-existing symptoms ("rebound phenomena"), anxiety, insomnia, restlessness, irritability, nausea, vomiting, stomach cramps, diarrhea, anorexia, weight loss, chills, and cold sweats, among others (Gallant et al., 1964; Gardos et al., 1978; Greenberg & Roth, 1966; Gualtieri, Quade et al., 1984).

In some publications, the reports on withdrawal symptoms are anecdotal (Gallant et al., 1964). Others used rating scales such as the Rating Scale for Chronic Schizophrenia by Lorr et al. (1953), and Wilcox's Gardner Behavior Chart (Greenberg & Roth, 1966).

Engelhardt developed the Withdrawal Emergent Symptom Checklist (WESC) (unpublished manuscript). This is a 13-item scale, with ratings of mild, moderate, and severe dyskinetic and other withdrawal symptoms. The 13 categories are as follows: choreoathetoid movements of limbs, head, trunk; myoclonic movements of limbs, head, trunk; lip-mouth movements, facial tics; posturing; tongue movements; disturbance of balance; terminal tremor; hypertonia; increased perspiration; vomiting; weight loss; anorexia; and euphoria, elation. Klein et al. (1980) and van der Kolk et al. (1978) are recommended for reviews of the literature.

Central Nervous System Side Effects

This group of side effects is commonly observed with all psychoactive drugs; some are dose related. Information is obtained by a variety of methods ranging from patient's history and physical/neurological examination, to subjective and objective global or multi-item rating scales, frequency counts, electromyography, tremography, and video-taping, among others. Clearly this is a very important area of research, and new, more reliable, valid, and objective measures are needed.

Extrapyramidal Side Effects

This group of side effects occurs with neuroleptic administration:

Acute dystonic reactions. These are prolonged and abnormal tonic contractions of muscles in the form of oculogyric crisis, torticollis, opisthotonus, and spasms of the tongue and of the torso. They are usually observed in the earliest stages of administration of neuroleptics and may last from a few minutes to several hours. There are no specific scales developed for these side effects; they are often included in other movement disorder scales (e.g., Crane & Naranjo, 1971).

Acute dyskinesias. These are among the earliest manifestations of extrapyramidal side effects seen with neuroleptics, as are the dystonias. The dyskinesias are clonic, involuntary spasms of muscle groups in the form of facial tics, blinking, chewing movements, lip smacking, tongue movements, shoulder shrugging, and pedaling of lower extremities. There are no specific scales in existence for these reactions; as in the case of the acute dystonic reactions, they are listed in movement disorder scales (e.g., Crane & Naranjo, 1971).

Parkinsonian reactions. They are usually seen in the first three weeks of treatment with neuroleptics. Akinesia, mask-like face, shuffling gait, finger and hand tremor, muscular rigidity, and drooling are most commonly observed.

The parkinsonian reactions were quantified in the Simpson-Angus Scale for Extrapyramidal Symptoms (SASEPS; Simpson & Angus, 1970). Each of ten operationally defined items is rated on a 5-point scale—0 meaning absence of the condition and 4 indicating its presence to an extremely severe degree. The validity and reliability of the scale were demonstrated. This revised scale represents an improvement over the earlier version (Simpson et al., 1964), as it includes two additional conditions: tremor and salivation. Instructions for administration are provided.

The Smith Tardive Dyskinesia Scale (in Fann et al., 1980) contains 11 items for parkinsonian reactions (regular tremor of tongue, salivation, regular tremor of eyes, no blinking of eyes, masked rigid facial expression, pill-rolling tremor of fingers, regular resting tremor of fingers, regular tremor of elbows and arms, diminished arm swing with arm rigid (not flaccid), regular tremor of leg and ankle tendon; and rigid, shuffling gait) to be rated on a 6-point scale from 0 (absent) to 5 (severe).

Akathisia. This occurs usually in the first 5 weeks of neuroleptic administration, but it may occur within 6 hours after 5 mg of oral haloperidol (Van Putten et al., 1984). Its manifestations are continuous agitation and restlessness, inability to sit still, and constant pacing. There is no specific scale for this condition, though it is contained in other scales, such as the one developed by Crane and Naranjo (1971).

Rabbit syndrome. This has a late onset and is a rare subcategory of extrapyramidal untoward effects. It is characterized by perioral muscular movements resembling the very rapid, chewing-like movements of the rabbit (Villeneuve, 1972). To the best of our knowledge, there is no specific scale for the assessment of this syndrome, although it has been included as an item in one general type of rating scale, the Smith Tardive Dyskinesia Scale (in Fann et al., 1980, pp. 247-254).

Other central nervous system side effects. These include excessive sedation, dizziness, headache, confusion, insomnia, depersonalization, ataxia, and grand mal seizures, among others. Many of these side effects are observed commonly after administration of all psychoactive agents.

For the assessment of central nervous system side effects, checklists for untoward effects are usually developed for specific drugs, such as the Lithium Toxicity Checklist for lithium (LTCL; Shopsin and Gershon, 1973, pp. 108-109). Some of these side effects are listed in more general side effect scales, such as the Dosage Record and Treatment Emergent Symptoms (DOTES), and the Subjects Treatment Emergent Symptom Scale (STESS), both developed by the Early Clinical Drug Evaluation Unit (ECDEU) of the Psychopharmacology Research Branch of the NIMH (Guy, 1976). The STESS is a 32-item scale, rated on 4 points: not at all (0), just a little (1), pretty much (2), very much (3). The scale is suitable for children up to age 15, and was designed to elicit information about the existence of various complaints, including physical ones. The child, parent, or a caretaker can complete the scale. Clearly, as with all studies of drug effects, it is essential that assessments be made during the baseline period, prior to drug administration.

Tardive and Withdrawal Dyskinesias

Tardive dyskinesia is one of the untoward manifestations of long-term neuroleptic treatment. It is an abnormal involuntary movement disorder most frequently involving the mouth, tongue, face, and extending to the neck, trunk, and extremities, even to the toes. It typically consists of slow and rhythmical movements of the facial and bucco-lingual-masticatory area, but can involve any part of the body in the form of myoclonic, athetotic or choreiform, dystonic, or tic-like movements. Respiratory dyskinesia due to abnormal diaphragmatic activity, and peculiar vocalizations and grunts also occur.

A variety of adjectives have been used to characterize these movements, such as "repetitive," "persistent," "irregular," "rhythmic," and "bizarre," to name a few. They disappear during sleep and they can be activated or temporarily suppressed by voluntary movements, tasks, or other muscle activities, and emotional factors.

This group of side effects has been classified as tardive dyskinesia, covert dyskinesia, and withdrawal dyskinesia (Crane & Naranjo, 1971; Gardos et al., 1978). In contrast to neuroleptic-induced parkinsonism, akathisia, acute dystonic reaction, and acute dyskinesia (the four other extrapyramidal system disorders), which almost always occur in the first hours, days, or weeks of drug treatment, tardive dyskinesia is usually seen months or years after starting neuroleptic administration. Whereas the above extrapyramidal reactions are reversible, tardive dyskinesia is thought to be irreversible in most cases. In addition, the early onset extrapyramidal side effects respond differently to treatment and to discontinuation of neuroleptics than the late onset group. The early onset group responds beneficially to dosage reduction, to treatment with antiparkinsonian agents (or, in the case of acute dystonic reaction, to diphenhydramine, given orally or intramuscularly) and is reversible by discontinuation of the neuroleptic. The opposite is true for tardive dyskinesia (for review, see Berger & Rexroth, 1980; Granacher, 1981). Actually, with the discontinuation of the neuroleptic, the so-called withdrawal dyskinesias may emerge (Gardos et al., 1978).

The significance of tardive dyskinesia in adult patients, and even in children, has been given increasing recognition in the past few years as evidenced by growing research (Berger & Rexroth, 1980; Campbell, Anderson et al., 1982; Campbell, Grega et al., 1983; Campbell, Perry et al., 1983; Gualtieri, Breuning et al., 1982; Gualtieri et al., 1980; Perry et al., 1985). However, the wide discrepancy of the prevalence of tardive dyskinesia (ranging from 0.5 percent to 57 percent in various reports) is indicative of the following: (1) lack of strict and agreed upon criteria in studies and reports, (2) lack of or difficulty in differentiating neuro-leptic-induced dyskinesias from such non-drug-induced dyskinesias as stereotyped movement disorders (American Psychiatric Association, DSM-III, 1980), stereotypies and posturings seen in nonmedicated schizophrenics, and stereotypies in infantile autism and mentally retarded individuals, among others, (3) lack of satisfactory (valid, reliable, and sensitive) assessment methods, (4) lack of accurate past drug history (this includes drug compliance, polypharmacy, usage of several neuroleptics over time), (5) patient variance, and (6) environ-mental variance (for review, see Gardos et al., 1977; Granacher, 1981; Berger & Rexroth, 1980; Kane & Smith, 1982; Schooler & Kane, 1982). The issues concerning assessment methods were critically reviewed by Gardos and associates (Gardos et al., 1977; Gardos & Cole, 1980a). The child literature was reviewed by Gualtieri et al. (1980), and Campbell, Grega et al. (1983).

There are no established and universally accepted criteria for the diagnosis of tardive dyskinesia (Gardos & Cole, 1980a; Schooler & Kane, 1982) especially in the milder or questionable cases. Perhaps this is the single most important problem concerning the assessment of tardive dyskinesia, a disorder that has become a major public health problem (Gardos & Cole, 1980b).

Assessment techniques include rating scales, frequency counts, instrumentation, and audio-visual methods (Gardos et al., 1977; Gardos & Cole, 1980a).

Rating scales can be divided into global rating scales and multi-item scales. Although global rating scales usually have good validity and require little training, their reliability is not always acceptable or is not reported. They can be "too global," at times assessing entire body parts rather than individual movements. The most frequently used scale of this type is the Abnormal Involuntary Movements Scale (AIMS), a standardized rating instrument developed by the Psychopharmacology Research Branch of the National Institute of Mental Health (NIMH). It has been employed both in adult and child populations (Campbell, Cohen et al., 1982; Campbell, Perry et al., 1983; Perry et al., 1985). The scale is organized into three groups of movements: facial and oral (muscles of facial expression, lips and perioral area, jaw, and tongue), extremity movements (upper and lower), and trunk movements (neck, shoulder, and hips). In addition, there are 3 items under the heading of global judgments (severity of abnormal movements, incapacitation due to abnormal movements, and patient's awareness of abnormal movements) and two under the heading of dental status (current problems with teeth or dentures, and whether patient usually wears dentures). Thus, there is a total of 12 items, measured on a 5-point scale (0, none; 1, minimal, may be extreme normal; 2, mild; 3, moderate; 4, severe). Tremor is not included in this scale, perhaps because tremor is rare in patients with marked tardive dyskinesia (Crane & Naranjo, 1971). Diagnostic criteria for possible subtypes, such as probable, masked probable, transient, withdrawal, persistent, and masked persistent tardive dyskinesia using the AIMS, or the Rockland Simpson Tardive Dyskinesia Rating Scale (in Fann et al., 1980) have been discussed by Schooler and Kane (1982).

A global rating scale specifically for the buccolingual-masticatory syndrome has been developed by Crane (Crane & Smeets, 1974); the severity of the disorder was measured on a 7-point scale (0, absent to 6, extremely severe). Other global scales have been reviewed by Gardos and associates (Gardos et al., 1977; Gardos & Cole, 1980a).

Multi-item rating scales are more detailed, with separate items for each abnormal movement, rather than for parts of the body. As with multi-item behavioral rating scales, the reliability may pose a problem.

Crane was the first to develop this type of scale for the rating of tardive dyskinesia; the scale has undergone various modifications. In one of the versions (Crane & Naranjo, 1971), tardive dyskinesia symptoms represent part of a 16-item rating scale, with items of abnormal motor disorders and postures in patients treated with neuroleptics. These tardive dyskinetic movements are as follows: complex dyskinesias (oculofacial type; bucco-lingual-mandibular type; of the upper extremities; of the lower extremities; and of the respiratory type), astasia, chorea, athetosis, dystonia, ballismus, postural disorders (in extension, in torsion; in lateral flexion), retrocollis, and other (e.g., ataxia). The first seven symptom clusters pertain to acute dystonia and dyskinesia, and various parkinsonian signs. The scale was used on approximately 100 hospitalized patients; a description of the items is given by the authors.

It was on the basis of Crane's scales that a 25-item scale, the Smith Tardive Dyskinesia Scale, was developed (in Fann et al., 1980, pp.

247-254) with 14 items for tardive dyskinesia and 11 items for parkinsonian symptoms. The items are well defined and their severity is rated on the following scale: 0, absent; 1, slight, doubtful; 2, mild; 3, moderate; 4, moderately severe; 5, severe. Ratings are done during a 5-10 minute structured observation. Instructions are provided. Interrater reliability was satisfactory; in one of the studies r = .80 to .95 on the total tardive dyskinesia score (Smith et al., 1977).

The Simpson Tardive Dyskinesia Rating Scale (in Fann et al., 1980, pp. 255-261) consists of 34 items, plus 6 "others" (to be described). They are organized under movement of face, neck and trunk, upper and lower extremities, and those of the entire body. The scale includes the rabbit syndrome, which is actually a late onset extrapyramidal symptom. The items are rated on a 6-point severity scale (1, absent; 2, possibly present; 3, mild; 4, moderate; 5, moderately severe; and 6, very severe). All items are defined.

The Abbreviated (Simpson) Dyskinesia Rating Scale (ADS) is an abridged form of the above 34-item scale (Simpson et al., 1979). It consists of 17 items, including 4 "others" to be described; this too is a 6-point instrument, providing clear-cut definition. Both instruments were developed for adult patients, though the ADS has been used in children (Campbell, Cohen et al., 1982; Campbell, Perry et al., 1983; Perry et al., 1985.) The Simpson Tardive Dyskinesia Rating Scale is a very comprehensive rating scale that has been widely used. Interrater reliability was 0.98 for the total score and for individual items from 0.55 to 0.99 (with a median of 0.91; Simpson et al., 1979).

The Gerlach Tardive Dyskinesia and Parkinsonism Rating Scale (in Fann et al., 1980, p. 267) consists of a three-part rating scale used for oral abnormal movements. The first item is a scale from 0 to 6 rating the frequency of the movement. In the second item, a scale from 0 to 6 measures in centimeters the amplitude of the abnormal movement, mouth opening and/or tongue protrusion. The third item measures in seconds (less than 1 second to more than 10 seconds) the duration of each tongue protrusion or mouth opening on a scale from 0 to 3. The scale is used twice during each evaluation (1) while the patient is unoccupied and undisturbed (passive) and (2) while the patient performs a specific voluntary task, such as drawing a spiral (active). The scale is carefully quantified for oral movements and is reported to be sensitive. Chien et al. (1980) report an interrater reliability correlation coefficient of 0.763 (p < 0.005) between two raters in their ratings of 38 dyskinetic patients. Apparently video recordings of the ratings should be used (Gerlach & Faurbye, 1980).

Counting the frequency of dyskinetic movements is another objective assessment method. So far it has only been tested on small samples but the method is sensitive enough to detect changes due to treatment (Kazamatsuri et al., 1973). The frequency count procedure was reviewed extensively by Gardos et al. (1977).

Methods measuring tardive dyskinesia with the aid of instruments include electromyography, electroencephalography, tremography, and electronic testing procedures based on accelerometer, among others; they were reviewed critically elsewhere (Gardos et al., 1977; Gardos & Cole, 1980a). Although these are the most precise and objective methods of assessment, their validity remains questionable and clinical usefulness is doubtful.

Vocal impairment in patients with tardive dyskinesia was measured by quantified assessment methods (Fann et al., 1977).

Videotaping is frequently used in studies of tardive dyskinesia; its main role is in research, education, and training (for review, see Gardos et al., 1977). Though high interrater reliability can be achieved with this method, the relationship between live and audio-visual rating methods has been shown only in one study involving 24 autistic children: The agreement was high (Perry et al., 1985).

Many central nervous system side effects, as well as some behavioral side effects, are contained in the Dosage Record and Treatment Emergent Symptom Scale (DOTES) developed by the Psychopharmacology Research Branch of the NIMH (Psychopharmacology Bulletin, 1973; ECDEU Assessment Manual, Guy, 1976), for both children and adults. One of the advantages of this scale is that dosage is readily related to side effects.

Supersensitivity Psychosis

It has been speculated that a neuroleptic-induced supersensitivity of mesolimbic dopamine receptors occurs in a subgroup of patients and manifests itself as insomnia, agitation, anxiety, and worsening of schizophrenic symptoms upon the withdrawal of neuroleptic (Chouinard & Jones, 1980). Clearly, this type of side effect can best be documented on a behavioral rating scale, with a stable pretreatment baseline, ratings throughout treatment, and during the withdrawal period.

In our research with autistic children over the past two decades, we have made the observation that behavior deteriorated in some children after neuroleptic withdrawal, and even became worse than it was on baseline; however, within a week or so, the symptoms returned to baseline level, or even decreased in severity to the same level as during neuroleptic treatment. We considered this to be a rebound phenomenon. Actually, some of these severely disturbed and impaired children were able to retain such gains as language and adaptive skills that they acquired during neuroleptic treatment (Campbell, Cohen et al., 1982). Only in one child have we observed phenomena comparable to supersensitivity psychosis in adults, namely the occurrence of insomnia, agitation, aggressiveness directed against others and self, and worsening of preexisting symptoms; they ceased within less than two weeks (Campbell, Grega et al., 1983). This child had follow-up psychological testing during this period and showed increases in adaptive (27-point increase), motor (10-point increase), and personal-social (17-point increase) developmental quotients (DQ) as measured by Gesell Developmental Schedules (Gesell & Amatruda, 1947); language DQ remained unchanged. In a retrospective study, Gualtieri, Quade et al. (1984) reported on this phenomenon, which they called "a behavioral analogue" of tardive dyskinesia, in mentally retarded and hyperactive youngsters.

Electrophysiological Side Effects

The use of the electroencephalogram (EEG) and sensory evoked potentials (EP) in psychopharmacology can be viewed as an attempt to correlate drug-induced electrophysiological changes to behavioral changes and to toxicity produced by the same drug. These attempts were not always successful (Fink, 1978; Shagas & Straumanis, 1978).

Heninger (1978) assessed the effects of lithium on behavior and brain function (quantified EEG, somatosensory, auditory, and visual cerebral-evoked response) in 18 patients, pre- and post-treatment. No placebo controls were employed. The median daily dose of lithium was 1,500 mg/d (dose range from 100 to 2,400 mg/d) with a median serum lithium of 1.1 mEq/l (ranging from 0.7 to 1.8 mEq/l). There was a significant increase of delta and theta intensity and a slowing of over 1 cps of the frequency of alpha peak during the lithium maintenance (9 to 62 days). The toxic increase of delta activity was observed in patients who showed behavioral worsening, which included lethargy, muscular tremor, nausea, and polyuria; they tended to occur at higher serum lithium levels. However, the other patients who had only minimal or no untoward effects showed the same type of EEG changes (possibly less marked) at somewhat lower serum lithium concentrations from 0.8 to 1.0 mEq/l.

In a small sample of severely disturbed children, ages 3 to 6 years, an attempt was made to relate clinical changes to EEG during lithium and chlorpromazine administration. There appeared to be a difference in therapeutic response in children whose baseline (predrug) EEGs showed focal abnormalities and those who had normal EEGs. If lithium accentuated the focal abnormality the behavior tended to worsen or to show no change (Campbell, Fish, Korein et al., 1972). However, if the focal abnormality of EEG was decreased by lithium, or if in the normal baseline EEG lithium produced changes such as diffuse slowing and slower alpha, behavioral improvement tended to occur. This relationship between focal EEG abnormality and behavioral change applied to both lithium and chlorpromazine.

EEG studies were conducted in a subsample of 61 children, diagnosed as conduct disorder, aggressive type, who were randomly assigned to lithium, haloperidol or placebo treatment under double-blind conditions (Campbell, Small et al., 1984). The EEG studies were completed on 44 boys and 4 girls and were carried out during the two-week baseline period and at the end of treatment during the optimal drug dose (Bennett et al., 1983). Two raters blind as to the patients' drug condition independently read the EEGs. Of the 48 children, 30 had abnormal EEG records on baseline, prior to drug administration. There was a significant probability ($p < 0.001$) that children who were receiving haloperidol or lithium had a worsening of the EEG records; this was not true for children who were assigned to placebo treatment (only 3 of the 16 children showed worsening of the EEG records). Comparing haloperidol alone to placebo, there was a significant probability that receiving haloperidol would result in worsening of the EEG record ($p < 0.05$); this was even more significant for lithium ($p < 0.001$). In general, the administration of either lithium or haloperidol tended to yield an increase in paroxysmal and focal abnormalities as compared to baseline; the severity of the abnormality was more pronounced with lithium than with haloperidol. However, administration of haloperidol was associated with the presence of more side effects—including effects at optimal dose—than was lithium, even though there were no statistical differences in their efficacy (Campbell, Small et al., 1984).

Autonomic Nervous System Side Effects

Autonomic nervous system side effects are observed with most classes of psychoactive drugs: neuroleptics, antidepressants, minor tranquilizers, and lithium. They include dry mouth, mydriasis, blurred vision, failure of accommodation, glaucoma, urinary retention, sweating, nausea, vomiting, dysphagia, paralytic ileus, constipation, diarrhea, and hypo- and hyperthermia, among others.

Some of these side effects are included in more general rating scales, such as the DOTES (hypotension, syncope/dizziness, tachycardia, nausea/vomiting, diarrhea). Investigators frequently develop their own side effect checklists in clinical trials for a specific drug, listing the autonomic side effects expected from the respective drug.

Careful clinical monitoring of these side effects is essential, as some of these side effects are potentially serious. However, often it is difficult to differentiate psychoactive drug-induced autonomic reactions from symptoms of the clinical entity for which the medication is prescribed. For example, severe depression is frequently associated with dry mouth and constipation and these are the most frequent side effects seen with antidepressant drugs. Thus, a stable baseline assessment is needed, including a detailed history and physical examination in order to establish what symptoms are part of the clinical pathology and which ones are adverse drug reactions.

The following readings are suggested: Belfer & Shader (1970); Klein et al. (1980); van der Kolk et al. (1978).

Cardiovascular Side Effects

Neuroleptics and particularly the tricyclic antidepressants are two classes of drugs that are especially associated with the production of cardiovascular side effects; these effects can also be associated with lithium administration. They are manifested as abnormalities of blood pressure, pulse, and electrocardiogram (EKG), including conduction changes. Some adult patients who receive psychoactive drugs have preexisting cardiovascular disease; thus particular caution is warranted in such cases. Little is known about the cardiovascular status of patient populations, such as schizophrenics, who do not receive psychoactive drugs. However, there is some, though inconclusive, evidence that certain EKG abnormalities—such as prolongation of Q-T interval—may be related to the pathophysiology of the illness, rather than being a drug side effect (Rainey, 1982).

A careful history and physical examination should precede treatment. The examination should include recordings of blood pressure and pulse; in certain instances such objective and quantified measures as EKG, echocardiogram (see Murburg et al., 1982), gated pool, and galium scanning are required with continuous monitoring throughout treatment. In children, regular EKG monitoring is recommended when imipramine does approach 5 mg/kg/day; investigational protocols for children will not be approved by the FDA if this dose is exceeded (Hayes et al., 1975).

Cardiovascular effects of psychoactive drugs, mainly of phenothiazines and antidepressants, were reviewed by Ebert and Shader (1970a), and of tricyclic antidepressants by Bigger et al. (1978).

Abnormal Laboratory Findings

Laboratory abnormalities can be associated with the administration of all drugs in the form of hematologic, blood chemistry, liver, and urine abnormalities. The Psychopharmacology Research Branch of the NIMH has developed a 52-item form, the Laboratory Data (LAB) for recording the data from various laboratory tests (*Psychopharmacology Bulletin,* 1973; Guy, 1976).

It has been pointed out that clinical laboratory data prior to drug administration (baseline) and their changes with drug treatment are part of assessment of the efficacy and safety of a new drug (Gershon, 1973). However, baseline laboratory values in certain patient populations may show variation from textbook normative data (Gershon, 1973; McGlashan & Cleary, 1975, 1976). Such patient populations may also show greater fluctuation in certain laboratory values over time without any drug administration than is expected in normals.

We have conducted a study in preschool age autistic children and made the observation that hematologic and liver profile values show great fluctuation in the same patient while on placebo maintenance (Campbell, unpublished data). Thus, norms are needed from special populations (e.g., schizophrenics, autistics, particularly in the pediatric age group) where textbooks often give vague values referring to adult norms and where maturational factors play a role (Gershon, 1973). In a recent review on tricyclic drugs it was pointed out that this class of drugs is known to cause false results: Spuriously elevated tests of liver functions, falsely low cholesterol values, and abnormal fasting blood sugar (Kessler, 1978) have been reported. Finally, quality control in the laboratory must be maintained in order to avoid errors.

Abnormal laboratory findings associated with psychotropic drug administration (hematologic and hepatic) were reviewed by Ebert and Shader (1970b, 1970c); those of tricyclics by Kessler (1978), and those of lithium by Gershon and Shopsin (1973), Reisberg and Gershon (1979),

Jenner (1979), and in children by Campbell, Perry et al. (1984); and Campbell, Small et al. (1984).

Endocrine and Metabolic Side Effects

Amenorrhea, gynecomastia, galactorrhea, thyroid gland and hormone changes, decrease of blood sugar, decrease or increase of plasma growth hormone level, lowering of plasma cortisol levels, and increase of prolactin are some of the endocrine effects of various classes of psychoactive drugs. Excessive weight gain is common in both adults and children with neuroleptics and tricyclics, whereas the psychomotor stimulants often cause a decrease of appetite and weight.

The problems and comments under the heading of laboratory toxicity are valid here. Not only do psychotropic drugs affect neurotransmitters and endocrine functions (Ganong & Martini, 1973; Kline, 1968; Martini & Ganong, 1971; Prange, 1974; Sachar, 1976), but stress and psychiatric disorders also affect neuroendocrine mechanisms (Campbell, Green et al., 1982; Carroll, 1978; Green, in press; Green, Campbell, & David, 1984; Green, Deutsch, & Campbell, in press; Prange, 1974; Shader & DiMascio, 1970). More carefully conducted research is needed in this area, perhaps involving large collaborative studies. Well-run laboratories with good quality control are essential for reproducible results.

Adverse Effects of Psychoactive Drugs on IQ

Monitoring of the IQ by standardized intelligence tests should be done on a yearly basis in those children and mentally retarded adults who require long-term drug administration because of their severe behavioral problems. Unfortunately, the interpretation of IQ data is not always clear-cut, for when the patient is institutionalized, adverse drug effects may be confused with the effects of chronic institutionalization itself. Most of the research concerning psychotropic drug effects on IQ was carried out in the mentally retarded. Little work has been done in children. The reader is referred to Aman (1978, 1984) for a review.

Though no particular assessment method was used, of the 24 artists treated on a long-term basis with lithium, 12 found that their creativity was increased by receiving the drug, 6 found no changes, and 6 felt that their productivity decreased (Schou, 1981).

Adverse Effects of Psychoactive
Drugs on Linear Growth

Tanner (1973) has reviewed the clinical essentials of the study of growth in children. He stresses the need to use modern, well-maintained equipment with a trained person making the measurements. For methods of measuring stature see Tanner et al., (1971, pp. 749-751). Puig-Antich, Greenhill et al. (1978) suggest the use of the Habner measuring table. It should be noted that, as with other variables or side effects that were discussed above, our knowledge is quite limited concerning growth in disturbed and retarded children (Campbell et al., 1980; Eggins et al., 1975; Roche et al., 1979; Simon & Gilles, 1964).

In the past 10 years there has been a concern over the possible adverse effects of psychoactive drugs, particularly the stimulants, on the growth of children. It started with the publication of a study by Safer and associates (1972) that had serious methodological flaws. McNutt and co-workers (1976) have presented a carefully planned and methodologically rigorous study. After one year, they found no significant differences in height and weight between 20 hyperactive children treated with a mean of 0.62 mg/kg methylphenidate and 23 normal controls. Their data did suggest, however, that hyperactive children, both medicated and nonmedicated, may have a different body composition from normal controls.

Roche et al. (1979) have noted that precise determination of the effects of stimulant medication on growth in children is difficult because of varying methodologies, designs, and accuracy of measurements. Nevertheless, it seems that stimulant drugs do produce slight to moderate growth suppression early in treatment, especially in the "high-normal" dose range. Weight is affected more than stature. Although the consensus is that tolerance develops and that eventual height and weight are not significantly affected, careful monitoring is especially advised for children who are small, and benefits versus risks must be weighed. Greenhill et al. (1980) suggest the stimulants may have differential growth suppression effects.

In some of the studies the growth charts employed were obtained from Boston and Iowa children in the 1930s. This has been corrected in a recent study by Mattes and Gittelman (1983), who employed recently updated growth charts in 86 hyperactive children receiving methylphenidate for up to 4 years. The growth norms were published in 1976 by the National Center of Health Statistics (Hamill et al., 1976). On these measures, there was a significant decrease in height and weight percentile on long-term methylphenidate administration (mean daily dose, 40 mg).

Carefully planned and methodologically rigorous studies, preferably large collaborative ones, are required to further clarify these important issues.

DIAGNOSIS

Careful diagnosis must precede treatment with psychoactive drugs, both in clinical trials and in "real-life" clinical practice. Diagnosis was difficult in the DSM (American Psychiatric Association, 1952) and DSM-II (American Psychiatric Association, 1968) era because clearcut diagnostic criteria were not given. DSM-III (American Psychiatric Association, 1980) represents a great improvement because it specifies inclusion and exclusion criteria, and frequently, duration of symptoms and time of onset of illness. This type of diagnostic system should help to facilitate communication between researchers by clearly identifying those patients or diagnostic subgroups who responded to a particular intervention. We have not yet attained the ideal of specific drugs for specific diagnostic categories, but we do know which classes of existing drugs are likely to be effective, and which of the existing drugs are contraindicated, for most psychiatric disorders in children.

DSM-III is already being revised, before adequate time has elapsed to assess its validity. Its relationship to the Ninth Revision of the International Classification of Diseases (ICD-9, 1977) and to pediatric psychopharmacology has been discussed by Gittelman-Klein et al. (1978). An excellent aid to DSM-III is a recent book by Rapoport and Ismond (1984).

Diagnosis alone is not sufficient for the development of a treatment plan in a child or adolescent: A profile of deficits (and assets) is required, and because deficits are often multiple, treatment for each should be specified. The clinician must then determine whether pharmacotherapy (and which specific drug) is indicated. Though ideally one should treat a disease entity or functions (Irwin, 1968), in many cases target symptoms are still being treated by pharmacotherapy. For example, the observation was made that autistic children, particularly those who are hypoactive, respond poorly to the sedative type, low potency phenothiazines, such as chlorpromazine (Campbell, Fish, Korein et al., 1972; Campbell, Fish et al., 1972), and that those who are hyperactive, normoactive, or in whom hyperactivity alternates with hypoactivity, respond well as a group to the high potency butyrophenone, haloperidol (Anderson et al., 1984). It has also been shown that schizophrenic adolescents respond better to thiothixene, a high-potency nonsedative neuroleptic (Realmuto et al., 1984).

INDICATIONS FOR PHARMACOTHERAPY

The decision to implement drug treatment must be based upon a sound diagnosis that includes an evaluation of the child's assets and deficits. Drug treatment should be reserved for those children whose symptoms are sufficiently severe as to impede normal emotional and social development or the ability to learn. Drug use should be viewed as part of a comprehensive program of treatment that frequently includes psychosocial, behavioral, and special educational interventions. The immediate and long-term side effects or evaluation of the risk-benefit ratio for an individual child must be considered prior to prescribing a specific medication. Depending upon the specific indication, pharmacotherapy should proceed at optimal dosages for periods of two and up to six months. After this time, the drug should be discontinued for about four weeks to permit evaluation of the need for continued treatment. Immediately following discontinuation, "rebound phenomena," usually due to cholinergic rebound or adrenergic activation, can occur. These withdrawal emergent symptoms are not an indication for resumption of drug therapy. Pharmacotherapy may be indicated in the following disorders:

Attention-deficit disorder with hyperactivity (ADDH). Psychomotor stimulants are the drugs of first choice in the management of ADDH in children 6 to 12 years of age. The superiority of these medications over placebo has been consistently shown in careful and controlled studies (for review, see Conners & Werry, 1979). In some stimulant-nonresponsive severely aggressive and hyperactive children, neuroleptics may be useful alternative agents.

Undersocialized conduct disorder, aggressive type. The salutary effects of short-term treatment with lithium or haloperidol in hospitalized, conduct disordered children who failed to respond to other interventions was recently shown (Campbell, Small et al., 1984). Thus pharmacotherapy for this highly prevalent disorder may be appropriate.

Schizophrenic and schizophreniform disorders. Although no controlled studies in prepubertal children exist, the nonsedative neuroleptics may be useful adjuncts in a total treatment program. Clinically, these drugs do not seem as effective in prepubertal patients as they do in adolescent and adult schizophrenic patients. In two controlled studies in adolescence, some neuroleptics were shown to be beneficial in reducing psychotic target symptoms (Pool et al., 1976; Realmuto et al., 1984).

Pervasive developmental disorders. In a series of systematic investigations of preschool age autistic children, haloperidol in a dosage range that does not cause sedation was shown to positively influence a variety of target symptoms (including stereotypies, hyperactivity, fidgetiness, withdrawal, and poor attention span) and to facilitate learning under controlled conditions (Anderson et al., 1984; Campbell, Anderson et al., 1978a). The existence and validity of childhood onset and atypical pervasive developmental disorders, as well as their relationship to infantile autism, are unknown. In those "atypical" children, nonsedating neuroleptics in relatively low dosages may be useful in the attenuation of target symptoms.

Affective disorders. Tricyclic antidepressants have not been approved for this indication in children under 12 years of age, but several well-controlled studies have shown that imipramine is effective in the treatment of prepubertal children who fulfill unmodified adult criteria for major depressive disorder (Puig-Antich et al., in press; Weller et al., 1983). Dosage should not exceed 5 mg/kg/day and cannot be used to predict therapeutic plasma levels. The role of tricyclics in the treatment of childhood disorders is still under investigation.

Stereotyped movement disorders. High potency neuroleptics, especially haloperidol, are indicated in the treatment of Tourette's disorder (Friedhoff & Chase, 1982) as well as other stereotyped movement disorders. Recently, pimozide, a novel neuroleptic of the diphenyl-butylpiperidine class that also binds to central calcium channels, has been approved for Tourette's disorder. Clonidine, a presynaptic alpha-adrenergic agonist that decreases central adrenergic tone, has been shown to reduce the severity of tics in Tourette's disorder. Stimulants are contraindicated in children with family histories of tics because they may precipitate the emergence of tics and Tourette's disorder in genetically predisposed individuals.

Disorders of sleep. Imipramine may be a useful intervention for the treatment of somnambulism and night terrors (Pessikoff & Davis, 1971).

These disorders may reflect an electrophysiologic disturbance of the deeper stages (stages 3 and 4) of sleep.

Functional enuresis. Imipramine is approved for use in the treatment of enuresis in children over the age of 6 years; a dosage of 2.5 mg/kg/day should not be exceeded. This drug should only be considered in the short-term or interim management of enuresis. Toxicity and the development of tolerance to the antienuretic effects, as well as the high rate of spontaneous remissions and existence of safe and effective alternative treatments, limit the long-term usefulness of this agent (Rapoport, Mikkelsen et al., 1980).

Behavioral symptoms associated with mental retardation. There have been few attempts to improve cognitive and intellectual performances in mentally retarded persons via pharmacological interventions. To date, pharmacological interventions have been aimed at the reduction of target symptoms, particularly hyperactivity, stereotypies, poor attention span, aggressiveness and self-injurious behaviors. Neuroleptics, especially thioridazine and chlorpromazine, have been most widely prescribed to control these symptoms. There are data to suggest that these drugs are effective in dosages of about half to several-fold lower than those that are usually prescribed (Singh & Aman, 1981). Moreover, in some patients, intellectual and workshop performance may actually improve following drug discontinuation. Stimulants are less effective in this population for the control of inattention, impulsivity, and hyperactivity (for review see Aman, 1984).

SPECIAL ISSUES FOR CHILDREN

Importance of Discussing Pharmacotherapy with Parents and Patient

If pharmacotherapy is indicated, after having discussed the child's diagnosis, condition, and entire treatment plan with the parents, the physician should review, in detail, the expected therapeutic benefits and possible untoward effects of the drug chosen. Some parents may be overly optimistic about the benefits of pharmacotherapy, whereas others may unrealistically view medication of the child as a shortcut for solving family problems. These issues must be dealt with in counseling sessions involving the parents alone or the entire family. Psychoactive drugs should not be prescribed on an outpatient basis unless the parents are reliable.

The children should be told why they are receiving medication in language appropriate to their cognitive abilities. They should be encouraged to ask questions and to express their feelings. If necessary, appropriate counseling can help to overcome a child's fears or worries about medication, including that it may take away his or her self-control. With the aggressive child, in particular, the physician should emphasize that medication alone will not resolve his or her problems; rather, medication will only assist the child with his or her own efforts to work on problems.

Dose Titration

The optimal therapeutic dose for many psychotropic medications is subject to wide interindividual variation among children. For some drugs, the optimal dose in pediatric patients is unrelated to weight, age, or illness severity. It is best to start with a low (perhaps therapeutically ineffective) dose and increase the dose gradually. In addition to behavioral observations of parents and teachers, the patient's subjective feelings and reactions to the medication should be elicited. Many children can verbalize their feelings when asked to do so. Thus they may report a sensation of being slowed down, irritable, or feeling calmer or more attentive at school once a therapeutic dosage has been attained. For younger or less verbal children, the clinician may have to rely more heavily on the reports of ward nurses, teachers, and parents.

A major error is to prescribe ineffectively low doses of a psychotropic medication. Underdosage exposes children to many of the risks but not the benefits of pharmacotherapy. At the other extreme, some clinicians give severely disturbed children an excessively high maintenance dose of drugs, usually neuroleptics. Unnecessary dose escalation can interfere with intellectual functioning and, in the case of neuroleptic, may hasten the development of tardive dyskinesia.

Whenever possible, the clinician should prescribe medication in a single daily dosage. This practice facilitates compliance and spares children the embarrassment of taking medication in front of school-mates. A single evening dose before sleep is not recommended, though there is disagreement on this point. With a single bedtime dosage schedule, behavioral and other effects occurring at peak blood levels may be missed and, in the case of neuroleptics, the risk of failing to recognize a serious acute dystonic reaction is increased.

Behavioral Toxicity

Children are more vulnerable than adults to behavioral toxicity from psychoactive drugs. Particularly in very young children, behavioral toxicity often precedes other treatment emergent symptoms such as parkinsonian side effects. Manifestations of behavioral toxicity can sometimes mimic the symptoms for which the drug was originally prescribed and are not an indication for an upward adjustment of dose. They include irritability, aggressiveness, and alteration of mood or activity level, among others. In order to recognize these symptoms as treatment emergent, careful monitoring of the patient is required during dosage regulation; they are managed by dose reduction. Although unknown, the increased occurrence of behavioral toxicity in young children could reflect central nervous system immaturity.

2

NEUROLEPTICS ✓

INDICATIONS

In child psychiatry neuroleptics are prescribed in a variety of disorders, whereas in adults they are used mainly for the treatment of schizophrenic and other psychotic disorders. Actually, schizophrenia and bipolar disorder are very rare in prepubertal children. As a rule, neuroleptics should be prescribed only to moderately to severely disturbed children, or for those who failed to respond to other types (or classes) of drugs. The various classes of neuroleptics and their representatives are listed in Table 1. Duration of treatment will vary from case to case. As a general rule, if the drug is effective, it should be given for at least 2 to 3 months (Gittelman-Klein, Klein, Katz et al., 1976). Drug treatment should be discontinued after 3 to 6 months (for about 4 weeks) in order to determine whether further drug administration is required, and whether withdrawal dyskinesias will develop (Campbell, Cohen et al., 1982; Campbell, Perry et al., 1983). After an initial rebound lasting for a few days, some children may no longer exhibit the behavioral symptoms for which the medication was initially prescribed.

The following are the conditions for which a trial of neuroleptic treatment is indicated, based on carefully conducted research, or on the basis of clinical experience:

Schizophrenic disorders. Little is known about the efficacy of neuroleptics in these conditions, though clinical experience indicates that these agents are less beneficial in children than in adults. Sedation is a major problem, and therefore it appears that the less sedative type of drugs, such as haloperidol, or thiothixene are of greater benefit (for review, Campbell, 1985).

Bipolar disorder, manic. In adults, haloperidol was reported to be effective in the treatment of mania (Shopsin et al., 1975). To the best of our knowledge, no information is available in children.

Infantile autism. It has been demonstrated that trifluoperazine and, particularly, haloperidol yield significant decreases of behavioral symptoms in certain young autistic children. Specifically, haloperidol, when administered over a period of 2 to 3 months to hyper- or normoactive patients in a structured educational/behavioral program, will enhance certain types of learning without untoward effects, if dosage is individually titrated (for review, see Campbell, Anderson et al., 1984).

Tourette's disorder. Haloperidol and pimozide appear to be the most effective agents in the treatment of this disorder (for review, see Friedhoff & Chase, 1982).

Conduct disorder, undersocialized, aggressive. Severe aggressiveness is usually unresponsive to stimulants, although some neuroleptics, particularly haloperidol, appear to be effective for reducing such maladaptive behavior (for review, see Campbell, Cohen et al., 1982).

Attention deficit disorder with hyperactivity. A trial of neuroleptic administration should be considered only in those patients who failed to respond to treatment with stimulants.

Mental retardation associated with behavioral symptoms. Aggressiveness directed against self or others and hyperactivity are the most common maladaptive behaviors in retarded youngsters. There is evidence that stimulants do not reduce these symptoms (Aman, 1984). A trial of neuroleptics is indicated only if behavioral approaches fail, though clinical experience has shown that in most cases aggressiveness is not responsive to this class of drugs, although cognition is usually adversely affected (for review, see Lipman et al., 1978; Sprague & Werry, 1971).

CONTRAINDICATIONS

Neuroleptics should not be prescribed to children with insomnia, or minor or reactive problems where behavioral measures and environmental manipulations are effective. Chlorpromazine is contraindicated in individuals with seizure disorder (Tarjan et al., 1957).

DOSAGE

Table 1 shows the dosage range of representative neuroleptics. However, it should be emphasized that individual dosage differences in children are great. Age, weight, and severity of symptoms will not necessarily determine the optimal therapeutic dose level for the individual child. Dosage should be individually titrated, starting with a low, usually ineffective dose. Increments should be gradual. By slow, gradual increments (even once a week) acute dystonic reactions can be avoided in most cases. Increments should be done at regular intervals, not more often than twice a week, until therapeutic effects occur. The

TABLE 1 Representative Neuroleptics and Dosages

Class of Neuroleptic	Generic Name (Trade Name)	CPZ Dose Equivalents*	Daily Dose Range (mg/day)	
			Children	Adolescents**
Phenothiazines				
(a) aliphatic	Chlorpromazine (Thorazine)	100	10-200 (maximum 2mg/kg)	—
(b) piperidine	Thioridazine (Mellaril)	100	10-200 (maximum 3mg/kg)	—
(c) piperazine	Trifluoperazine (Stelazine)	5	1-15	—
Butyrophenones	Haloperidol (Haldol)	1.6	0.5-16 (0.02-0.2mg/kg)	2-16 (mean 9.8)
Thioxanthenes	Thiothixene (Navane)	5	—	5-42 (mean 16.2)
Dibenzoxazepines	Loxapine (Loxitane)	10	—	20-100 (mean 87.5)
Dihydroindolones	Molindone (Moban)	6-10	—	1-40
Diphenylbutyl-piperidine	Pimozide (Orap)	—	1-4	1-4

*Chlorpromazine dose equivalents in mg; adapted from Davis (1985).
**If dosage is different than in children. Severely disturbed adolescents may require higher doses.

clinician should not exceed well established upper limits recommended by the Physician's Desk Reference (1985). The aim is to achieve a marked therapeutic effect without accompanying untoward effects, or with only minimal untoward effects that do not interfere with the patient's functioning at school and at home. There is supportive evidence that, under careful monitoring, diagnosis may be a factor determining whether therapeutic doses will or will not yield untoward effects. In preschool age autistic children, therapeutic doses of haloperidol (0.019 to 0.217 mg/kg/day; Anderson et al., 1984) resulted in no untoward effects. At comparable doses (0.04 to 0.21 mg/kg/day), excessive sedation and drooling occurred in school aged children of normal intelligence diagnosed as conduct disorder, aggressive type (Campbell, Small et al., 1984).

SHORT- AND LONG-TERM EFFICACY

Effect on Behavioral Symptoms

Hyperactivity, aggressiveness, temper tantrums, tics, stereotypies, withdrawal, hallucinations, and delusions are the symptoms that most commonly respond to neuroleptic administration.

Of the phenothiazines, chlorpromazine and thioridazine are the most frequently prescribed drugs: Both yield sedation, often at therapeutic doses. In outpatients of normal intellectual functioning characterized as hyperactive, chlorpromazine was shown to be an effective drug in reducing hyperactivity (Werry et al., 1966), though in some respects it was less effective than dextroamphetamine (Rapoport et al., 1971). In a large sample of children (N = 155) of similar behavioral profile, also treated in a clinic, thioridazine was compared to methylphenidate and to the combination of both drugs (Gittelman-Klein, Klein, Katz et al., 1976). It was hoped that the combination of a stimulant and a phenothiazine would increase the therapeutic effects because the two drugs have different profiles. It was also hoped that each would antagonize the side effect of the other. Treatment effects were evaluated at 4 and 12 weeks.

Methylphenidate and the combination of methylphenidate and thioridazine were superior to the administration of thioridazine alone; whereas methylphenidate seemed to yield increasing efficacy over time, the opposite was true for thioridazine. The combination of the two drugs showed only a trend of superiority over methylphenidate at week four, although at week 12 there was no difference between the two treatments. Hence, this study seems to establish the superiority of a stimulant over a phenothiazine in hyperactive children, because thioridazine caused enuresis, appetite increase, and excessive sedation, which interfered with daily functioning. It is noteworthy that 5 percent of the children did not require medication after 3 months of treatment. All three of the above studies were conducted under double-blind and placebo-controlled conditions, using a variety of rating scales and multiple raters.

In young autistic children, chlorpromazine did not yield marked improvement and was associated with excessive sedation (Campbell, Fish, Korein et al., 1972; Campbell, Fish, Shapiro et al., 1972). On the other hand, administration of trifluoperazine—a phenothiazine with a less sedative action than either chlorpromazine or thioridazine—resulted in a decrease of withdrawal and increases in alertness and verbal production in low functioning autistic children (Fish et al., 1966). In the same study, the higher-functioning patients responded to psychosocial treatments or showed worsening on the drug. In uncontrolled trials, fluphenazine was reported to decrease a variety of symptoms in both inpatient (Faretra et al., 1970) and outpatient (Engelhardt et al., 1973) autistics. Even though the age range of patients was the same in both studies, there was a great discrepancy in the dosages used: The inpatients received 0.75 to 3.75 mg of fluphenazine per day, whereas the mean dose in outpatients was 10.4 mg/day.

Thioridazine was studied only in a small sample of schizophrenic adolescents: Though the study has some methodological problems including small sample size, it is an important one as there is very little information about the efficacy of neuroleptics in this age group. In addition, the sample was diagnostically homogeneous and well defined. Patients were randomly assigned to thioridazine or thiothixene. Eight of the patients, ages 13 years, 9 months to 18 years, 9 months (mean, 16 years, 1 month) received thioridazine, mean daily dose of 3.3 mg/kg (or range of 91-228 mg/day, mean 178 mg/day) over a period of 4 to 6 weeks. There was a significant decrease of symptoms as measured on the Brief Psychiatric Rating Scale (BPRS); improvement was also rated on the Clinical Global Impressions Scale (CGI) from baseline to post-treatment (Realmuto et al., 1984). However, only half of the children showed improvement. This study confirms clinical impressions that the youngest schizophrenics are least responsive to treatment with neuroleptics, and that the youngest psychiatric patients, irrespective of diagnosis, show excessive sedation on low-potency neuroleptics, such as thiorida-zine, at doses where there is only little clinical improvement.

All the above studies report on the results of short-term administration of phenothiazines; little is known about the long-term efficacy of these drugs, even though they are often prescribed over long periods of time, particularly to retarded persons (Lipman et al., 1978). This practice may result in serious adverse effects, including tardive or withdrawal dyskinesias (Gualtieri, Breuning et al., 1982; Gualtieri, Quade et al., 1984).

In two large-scale retrospective studies involving heterogeneous samples of over 500 hospitalized mentally retarded persons, chlorproma-zine and thioridazine were reported to be effective in the amelioration of several target behaviors: hyperactivity, temper tantrums, self-injurious behaviors, aggressiveness toward others, and feeding difficulties includ-ing emesis (Pregelj & Barkauskas, 1967; Tarjan et al., 1957). According to the global impressions of physicians and staff, about 70 percent to 80 percent of the retarded patients responded favorably to these two medications. In fact, in one of the studies, involving 320 subjects (141 were between the ages 1 to 19 years) who were on neuroleptic maintenance for one year, medication was felt to reduce social withdrawal and to facilitate establishment of therapeutic relationships in some cases (Tarjan et al., 1957).

In the report of Pregelj and Barkauskas (1967) the majority of subjects showed global improvement on thioridazine, after 4 years of maintenance; of the 68 individuals who had seizure disorder, and who were receiving antiepileptics in addition to thioridazine, 60 (88.2 percent) showed a marked decrease in the frequency of the seizures. In contrast, chlorpromazine seemed to increase seizures significantly in 12 retarded individuals, though in 10 of the 12 phenobarbital was decreased or discontinued (Tarjan et al., 1957).

Due to the retrospective design and absence of double-blind proce-dures and standardized assessment instruments, two criticisms of these early studies naturally arose: First, that the positive therapeutic effects were due to nonspecific suppression of behaviors, including adaptive behaviors; and second that the results reflected investigator bias due to staff enthusiasm with the administration of relatively novel drugs to a new category of patient. A double-blind, placebo-controlled study involving 19 severely retarded institutionalized patients (14 males and 5 females; mean age 15.8 years) was designed to assess specific behavioral and other effects of thioridazine (Singh & Aman, 1981). Charge nurses

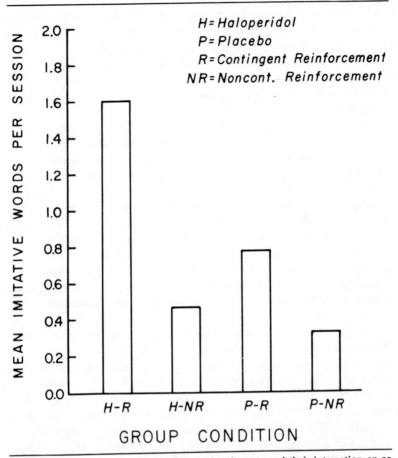

Figure 1: The effects of haloperidol, behavior therapy, and their interaction on acquisition of imitative speech in 40 autistic children ages 2.6 to 7.2 years.

evaluated drug efficacy with the CTQ and a four-point rating scale that assessed dimensions of appearance, screaming, self-injury, stereotyped movements, and bizarre behavior. In addition, the study included a comparison of individually titrated optimal doses (mean 5.23 mg/kg/day) with a "low" standardized dose (2.5 mg/kg/day). In general, pediatric house officers titrated individualized doses according to global assessments provided by the nursing staff. The authors felt that this procedure represents the common mode of dosage regulation in most institutions. Individualized doses ranged up to seven times greater than the standardized dose. Patients rotated through one of three possible sequences; each sequence included three four-week medication conditions: placebo, standardized dose, and individually titrated dose. Thioridazine administered over 6 months had beneficial effects on hyperactivity, stereotypic and self-stimulating behaviors, and bizarre behaviors without any significant alteration of other categories of behavior. Although tentative, the data are consistent with specific effects of thioridazine on these classes of behavior. Moreover, the data support a clinical role for thioridazine in carefully selected patients. The authors acknowledge that individual patients differ in their response to medication; however, the results of this study indicate that individually titrated dosages may be significantly higher than those necessary to achieve symptom reduction. Specifically, the relatively low standardized dose and the individualized doses were shown to be equally beneficial. Although dosages should continue to be individually regulated in mentally retarded populations, 2.5 mg/kg/day of thioridazine is a useful guideline for selection of optimal therapeutic dose. Optimal dosage should be the lowest therapeutically effective dose that is devoid of side effects.

Antipsychotic drugs with a high degree of antimuscarinic, antiadrenergic, and antihistaminic activity, such as chlorpromazine and thioridazine can result in cognitive dulling, impaired arousal, and sedation (for review, see Deutsch & Campbell, 1984). These side effects would interfere with the ability of patients to benefit from psychoeducational interventions and they are particularly troublesome in an already intellectually impaired population. Moreover, research data suggest that intellectual and workshop performance of some mentally retarded persons may actually improve following withdrawal from neuroleptics. Therefore, in the selection of a neuroleptic for retarded patients, it is probably best to prescribe a high-potency neuroleptic because these agents have relatively high affinity for dopaminergic receptors, but low affinity for cholinergic or adrenergic receptors. Furthermore, these agents should be prescribed in the smallest possible dose. The clinician should be alert for the emergence of neuroleptic induced abnormal involuntary movements involving the fingers, hands, and upper extremities because impairment of fine motor coordination could interfere with workshop performance and similar vocational-rehabilitation programs.

Weiss et al. (1979) found that hyperactive children who received chlorpromazine from 18 to 48 months did not differ from those who received drug for less than 6 months, when seen for follow-up 10 years later.

Haloperidol was explored and its efficacy assessed in a variety of conditions. It was found to be effective in both in- and outpatients with symptoms of aggressiveness and hyperactivity (Campbell, Cohen et al., 1982; Campbell, Small et al., 1984; Cunningham et al., 1968; Werry & Aman, 1975; Werry et al., 1975).

In 24 hyperactive or aggressive undersocialized children, haloperidol was administered in a crossover design, in high (0.05 mg/kg/day) and in low (0.025 mg/kg/day) doses (Werry & Aman, 1975). Assessments of these outpatients were made by various raters: Both doses of haloperidol were superior to placebo and they were as effective as methylphenidate (0.3 mg/kg/day) in decreasing the target symptoms.

In a more severely disturbed sample of children of the same age range (5 to 12 years), diagnosed as conduct disorder, undersocialized, aggressive, and hospitalized because they failed to respond to outpatient treatments, haloperidol administration resulted in significant decreases of aggressiveness, explosiveness, hyperactivity, and symptoms of hostility and negativism (Campbell, Small et al., 1984). The optimal doses employed ranged from 1.0 to 6.0 mg/day (mean 2.95) or 0.04 to 0.21 mg/kg/day (mean 0.096), and were higher than those used by Werry and his associates. This could be a function of severity of symptoms or of the condition itself. The study was double-blind and placebo-controlled; the children were rated under a variety of conditions independently by several raters. This was a short-term study.

In a similar population of outpatients, haloperidol (0.05 mg/kg/day) remained clinically effective when given over a period of 6 months (Wong & Cock, 1971). Children who were receiving placebo had a fluctuating course with only a statistical trend for haloperidol's superiority over placebo.

In schizophrenic inpatients (with acute schizophrenia, or acute exacerbation of chronic schizophrenia), ages 13 to 18 years, haloperidol (in doses of 2-16 mg/day, mean 9.8) was as effective as loxapine (in doses of 10-200 mg/day, mean 87.5) and both drugs were statistically superior to placebo in reducing various psychotic symptoms in a double-blind study (Pool et al., 1976). Well-designed studies are not available in prepubertal schizophrenic children, perhaps because the condition is quite rare (Green, Campbell, Hardesty et al., 1984; Kydd & Werry, 1982). As noted above, clinical experience suggests that young schizophrenics, unlike their older counterparts, are less responsive (or even nonresponsive) to pharmacotherapy.

There are two uncontrolled studies of haloperidol in autistic children (Engelhardt et al., 1973; Faretra et al., 1970). These led to more rigorous trials. Thus, haloperidol was compared to behavior therapy and to the combination of both modalities with respect to their effect on behavioral symptoms and on language acquisition, employing a between-groups design and a variety of rating scales (Campbell, Anderson et al., 1978). Haloperidol significantly reduced stereotypies and withdrawal in those children who were 4.5 years of age and older. The combination of haloperidol and behavior therapy (focusing on language acquisition) was significantly superior to other treatments in facilitating language acquisition in the laboratory. In a subsequent study, the efficacy of haloperidol was replicated in a within-subjects reversal design utilizing different rating scales (Cohen et al., 1980). From the first study involving 40 autistic children, ages 2.6 to 7.2 years, it was learned that haloperidol in combination with language therapy facilitates language acquisition as shown in Figure 1 (Campbell, Anderson et al., 1978). However, how this was achieved remained unanswered. Did haloperidol facilitate learning by decreasing stereotypies and withdrawal, so that the child could attend better to the behavior therapist, or did haloperidol facilitate learning by directly affecting some attentional mechanisms?

In order to answer this question a study was designed to assess in a large sample of autistic children the effects of haloperidol on behavioral symptoms, in two naturalistic environments (using multiple rating scales), in a highly structured experimental setting, and on learning (Anderson et al., 1984). In the highly structured experimental setting—a computer-controlled laboratory—the effects of haloperidol were assessed on behavioral symptoms (stereotypies, hyperactivity, and general motor activity) and on discrimination learning, employing an automated operant conditioning paradigm. A within-subjects reversal design was used, in which children were randomly assigned to one or the other treatment schedule: haloperidol-placebo-haloperidol, or placebo-halo-peridol-placebo (A1-B-A2), each treatment lasting for 4 weeks. The 40 autistic children, ages 2.33 to 6.92 years, showed the following response. Outside of the laboratory, there were significant decreases in ratings of stereotypies, withdrawal, hyperactivity, fidgetiness, abnormal object relationships, negativism, labile affect, and irritability during halo-peridol treatment, as shown in Figure 2. In the laboratory discrimination learning increased significantly during haloperidol treatment (Figures 3 and 4). Patients receiving haloperidol performed as well as patients on placebo who scored 20 points higher on Gesell Language Developmental Quotient. Of the children receiving haloperidol, 71

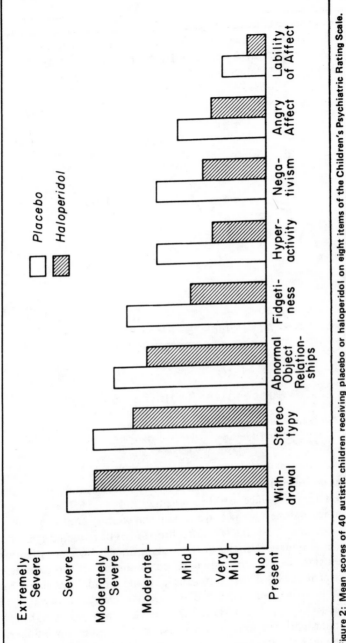

Figure 2: Mean scores of 40 autistic children receiving placebo or haloperidol on eight items of the Children's Psychiatric Rating Scale. (From Anderson et al., 1984, *American Journal of Psychiatry*; reprinted with permission.)

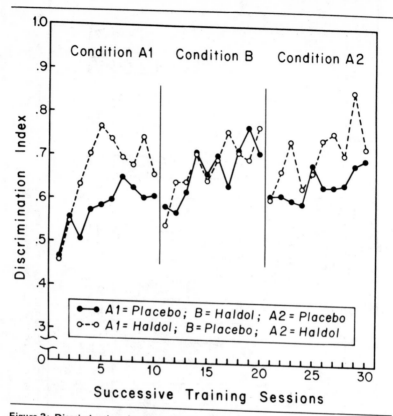

Figure 3: Discrimination learning in 32 autistic children during treatment with haloperidol or placebo. (From Anderson et al., 1984, *American Journal of Psychiatry*; reprinted with permission.)

percent performed at 0.6 criterion level, whereas only 39 percent of the children receiving placebo did so, as shown in Figure 5. However, in the laboratory, haloperidol had no effect on behavioral symptoms. Thus the effect of drug on learning was not a function of its reducing symptoms. One can speculate that the drug exerts a direct effect on attentional mechanisms, which are known to be abnormal in this population (Kolko et al., 1980). The optimal dosage of haloperidol was comparable to the two earlier controlled studies, though somewhat lower: 0.5 to 3.0 mg/day (mean 1.11) or 0.019 to 0.217 mg/kg/day (mean 0.05).

Autistic children were able to sustain their gains on haloperidol maintenance therapy on a long-term basis (at the 6-month follow-up

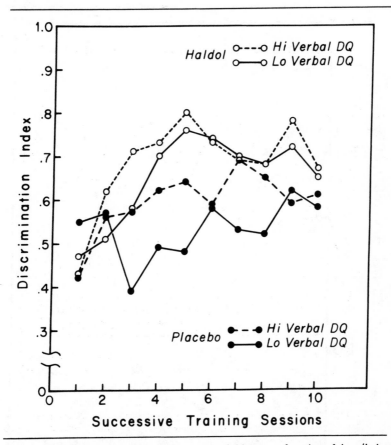

Figure 4: Discrimination learning in 32 autistic children as a function of drug (haloperidol or placebo) and language development quotient (DQ) in treatment
condition A1. (From Anderson et al., 1984, *American Journal of Psychiatry*, reprinted with permission.)

rating); one week after its discontinuation, stereotypies, withdrawal,
hyperactivity, fidgetiness, and abnormal object relations showed significant worsening as rated on the CPRS, and so did ratings on the CGI
(Campbell, Perry et al., 1983).

Haloperidol, in conservative doses (0.5 to 8.0 mg/day), is perhaps
one of the best treatments for Tourette's disorder: About 50 percent to
82.5 percent of patients show a reduction of tics (for review, see
Friedhoff & Chase, 1982). In a 7-month and up to 8.5-year follow-up,

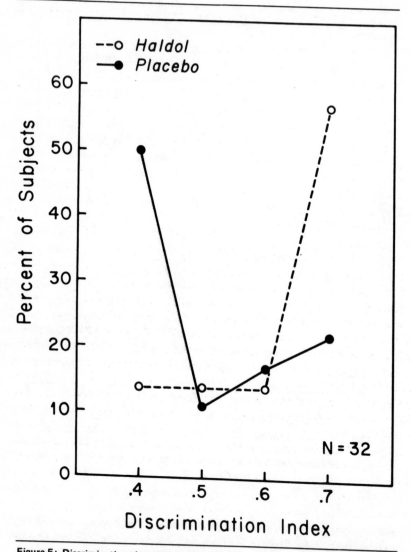

Figure 5: Discrimination learning in 32 autistic children receiving haloperidol or placebo: Frequency distribution as a function of discrimination indices in treatment condition A1. Discrimination indices scores are grouped as follows: .4 represents all scores below .5, .5 represents all scores between .5 and .59, .6 represents all scores between .6 and .69, and .7 represents all scores equal to or greater than .7. (From Anderson et al., 1984, *American Journal of Psychiatry;* reprinted with permission.)

the majority of patients retained their improvement on haloperidol maintenance (Shapiro & Shapiro, 1981).

Thiothixene, a member of the thioxanthene class of neuroleptics, was studied in schizophrenic and autistic patients: All reports consist of small sample sizes and none uses a placebo control. In the study by Realmuto et al. (1984) cited above, 21 chronic schizophrenic inpatients, ages 11 years and 9 months to 18 years and 9 months, were randomly assigned to thiothixene or to thioridazine after a baseline assessment. Thirteen of these patients (mean age 15 years 1 month) received thiothixene in daily doses ranging from 4.8 to 42.6 mg (mean 16.2 mg) or 0.30 mg/kg for a period of 4 to 6 weeks. Optimal dosage was determined individually and it was reached after about 2 weeks of regulation. The greatest reductions in symptoms of hallucinations, anxiety, tension, and excitement were within the first week of treatment, as rated on the BPRS; cognitive disorganization showed more gradual reduction. Changes were significant on both BPRS and on CGI from baseline to drug maintenance; however, only half of the sample showed improvement. There was no difference between the two drugs with respect to therapeutic efficacy.. However, there were fewer untoward effects from thiothixene than thioridazine: 6 of the 8 patients on thioridazine were drowsy, whereas only 7 of the 13 patients receiving thiothixene had this untoward effect. The authors conclude that, in general, young schizophrenics appear to be similar to adults with process schizophrenia and show poor response to neuroleptic treatment; and that high-potency neuroleptics such as thiothixene may be more beneficial in the treatment of these patients, because they are associated less frequently with excessive sedation than the low-potency neuroleptics.

Similar conclusions were made on the basis of two small pilot studies conducted in preschool age autistic children (Campbell et al., 1970; Fish et al., 1969). However, in this population, unlike in the schizophrenic adolescents, thiothixene had a wide therapeutic margin: At therapeutic doses ranging from 1 to 6 mg/day, only positive effects were rated; untoward effects developed at doses that were 1.3 to 6 times higher than the optimal dose (Campbell et al., 1970). Other reports involving thiothixene in children are those of Simeon and colleagues (1973), Waizer et al. (1972), and Wolpert et al. (1967).

Molindone, a dihydroindolone, was explored in infantile autism (age range 3 to 5 years, optimal dose 1-1.25 mg/day; Campbell et al., 1971) and in conduct disorder, aggressive (age range 6 to 11 years, optimal dose 18 to 155 mg/day, mean 40.5; Greenhill et al., 1981). Both are preliminary studies with promising findings; molindone warrants systematic and careful studies in children because it appears to have a wide therapeutic margin.

The efficacy of loxapine, a dibenzoxazepine, was demonstrated in schizophrenic adolescents (acute schizophrenia, or acute exacerbation of chronic schizophrenia) in a double-blind and placebo-controlled study (Pool et al., 1976) in which 75 inpatients, ages 13 to 18 years, were randomly assigned to loxapine, haloperidol, or placebo, after baseline assessments on the BPRS and Nurse's Observation Scale for Inpatient Evaluation (NOSIE). Loxapine, in daily doses of 10 to 200 mg (mean 87.5) was significantly superior to placebo, though it was more sedative than haloperidol.

Pimozide, a diphenylbutylpiperidine, is an effective drug (1.0 to 2.0 mg/day and up to 4 mg/day) in decreasing vocal and motor tics in Tourette's disorder (for review, see Friedhoff & Chase, 1982). It seems that pimozide is less sedative and has fewer extrapyramidal side effects than haloperidol at therapeutic doses (Debray et al., 1972; Messer-schmitt, 1972; Ross & Moldofsky, 1977; Shapiro & Shapiro, 1982, 1984), though this awaits confirmation.

Pimozide was also explored in psychotic children; however, the samples were diagnostically heterogeneous. Pangalila-Ratulangi (1973) reported clinical improvement without toxicity in 10 children diagnosed as having schizophrenia or schizophrenia-like symptomatology, at daily doses of 1 to 2 mg. In a multicenter study, pimozide (1-4 mg/day) was compared to haloperidol (0.75 to 6.75 mg/day) in a double-blind and placebo-controlled study (Naruse et al., 1982). The 87 patients, ages 3 to 16 years, were randomly assigned to one of the three treatments. A crossover design was used, but there was no washout at switchover. On global ratings, there was no difference between haloperidol and pimozide and both were superior to placebo. However, on behavioral rating scales, pimozide was more effective than haloperidol. The patients were diagnostically heterogeneous; 34 were autistic.

Effect on Cognition

There is a general belief that neuroleptics have an adverse effect on cognitive functions because of their tranquilizing sedative effects. This is supported by studies conducted in institutionalized mentally retarded individuals; these patients usually receive the sedative type of neurolep-tics such as the low-potency thioridazine or chlorpromazine (for review, see Lipman et al., 1978).

Only a few studies were conducted in carefully diagnosed children of normal intelligence. Werry et al. (1966), in a placebo-controlled double-blind clinical trial of chlorpromazine first involving 39 hyperactive outpatients (mean age 8.5 years) and later expanding the sample to 48, found that chlorpromazine (mean daily dose 106 mg) administration resulted in a trend toward improvement on the Continuous Performance Test, suggestive deterioration on the WISC comprehension subtest and on the Bender Gestalt orientation quotient, in the laboratory, after 8 weeks of treatment. The authors concluded that chlorpromazine is effective in reducing hyperactivity and improving attention, but that it has a slight depressant effect on cognition in the laboratory, in a one-to-one test situation.

Chlorpromazine (100-200 mg/day) had no effect on a cognitive battery administered to 4 hospitalized children, diagnosed as conduct disorder, with a behavioral profile of severe aggressiveness and explosiveness (Campbell, Cohen et al., 1982).

Haloperidol in daily doses of 0.05 mg/kg/day did not have an adverse effect on a battery of tasks measuring scholastic achievement and intellectual functioning in outpatient children with severe behavior disorders, when administered over a period of 6 months (Wong & Cock, 1971). Actually, there were significant increases of IQ in the 28 children who constituted the sample, irrespective of whether they received haloperidol or placebo. Cunningham et al. (1968) found psychomotor slowing in a group of 12 aggressive inpatients, ages 7 years, 8 months to 12 years, 10 months, on daily doses of 3.0 mg of haloperidol, or 0.08-0.12 mg/kg. This was a double-blind and placebo-controlled study.

Werry and Aman (1975) designed a study to determine whether the alleged adverse effect of neuroleptics on cognition is an effect of neuroleptic per se, or a function of dose. Haloperidol, both high dose (0.05 mg/kg/day) and low dose (0.025 mg/kg/day) was administered to 24 children, ages 4 years, 11 months to 12 years, 4 months, and compared to methylphenidate. In this double-blind, placebo-controlled crossover study, the subjects were hyperactive and aggressive outpatients, all of normal intelligence. The measures of cognitive function included a short-term recognition memory task (STM) and continuous performance task (CPT) with dependent variables as follows: the number of errors of omission, the number of errors of commission, the response time, and the number of seat movements. Low dose of haloperidol significantly reduced the number of false responses on the CPT compared with placebo and high dose of haloperidol, whereas methylphenidate was significantly superior to high dose of haloperidol on several measures, both on STM and on the CPT, when administered over a period of three weeks. Thus under these conditions, the adverse effect on cognitive functions appears to be a function of haloperidol dosage.

When given to a more severely disturbed population of inpatients, and in higher doses (mean 0.096 mg/kg/day; range 0.04 to 0.21 mg/kg/day), haloperidol administration was associated with significant decreases in Porteus Maze test quotient scores and a slowing of reaction time (RT) on a simple task (Platt et al., 1984). No significant drug effects were found on the Matching Familiar Figure Test, concept attainment tasks, short-term recognition memory, and on the Stroop Test in these 20 treatment-resistant patients diagnosed as conduct disorder (under-socialized, aggressive) with a behavioral profile of aggressiveness and explosiveness. Though the effects of haloperidol on cognition were mild, these findings seem to be in agreement with those of Werry and Aman (1975). It is noteworthy that in both studies haloperidol had significantly reduced behavioral symptoms (Campbell, Small et al., 1984; Werry et al., 1975).

In contrast to the depressant effects of haloperidol on cognitive functions in aggressive and hyperactive children of normal intelligence, haloperidol facilitated learning in the laboratory, when administered to preschool age autistic children. In mean doses of 0.07 mg/kg/day for children below, and 0.15 mg/kg/day for those above 4.5 years of age, haloperidol facilitated language acquisition when combined with lan-guage therapy; at these doses there were no effects on a cognitive battery (Campbell, Anderson et al., 1978). This drug also facilitated dis-crimination learning in autistic children ages 2.33 to 6.92 years at mean doses of 0.05 mg/kg/day (range 0.019 to 0.122 mg/kg/day; Anderson et al., 1984).

One can speculate that the adverse effects of haloperidol are not only a function of dose, but also a function of diagnosis, though the subjects diagnosed as conduct disorder in the Platt et al. (1984) study received higher doses as a group than the autistic children in the studies of Campbell, Anderson et al. (1978) and Anderson et al. (1984).

The effects of haloperidol on cognitive functions were assessed in a sample of children diagnosed as Tourette's disorder who were of normal intelligence. The 16 subjects, ages 7 to 21 years (mean 12 years, 4 months) were receiving haloperidol "for several months" (Bogomolny et al., 1982, p. 427) in daily doses of 0.5 to 3.0 mg or 0.009 to 0.122 mg/kg (mean 0.043). A crossover within-subjects design was employed; the two conditions were haloperidol or no drug in a random schedule. On-drug testing was done when the patient was receiving the optimal dose of haloperidol for at least 2 weeks; off-drug testing was carried out following a minimum of six days after drug discontinuation. Eighteen dependent variables making up eight tasks were employed: there were no significant adverse effects of haloperidol on higher cognitive functions involving planning, attention and memory, simple sensory and motor functions, and visual-motor integration. Patients made more qualitative errors on the enlarged Porteus mazes while off haloperidol (Bogomolny et al., 1982).

The effects of long-term administration of haloperidol on the intellectual functioning of autistic children, all of whom were functioning on subnormal levels, were assessed using a prospective design (Die Trill et al., 1984). Fifteen autistic children, ages 3.3 to 8.11 years, were retested after haloperidol (0.5 to 3.0 mg/day, mean 1.313) maintenance (mean 2 years). In eight children, there were increments in scores; in two, the scores remained stable; and in five children there was decrement in functioning. These results have to be interpreted with caution, because no controls were used. However, follow-up data indicate that in infantile autism IQs have predictive value and they maintain moderate stability throughout middle childhood and adolescence (Lockyer & Rutter, 1969).

The effects of long-term phenothiazine maintenance were assessed in a large sample of institutionalized children on a variety of measures (McAndrew et al., 1972). After discontinuation of drug administration, significant increases in scores on the Stanford Achievement battery were obtained in three children. These aggressive and nonpsychotic patients, ages 12 to 13 years—who were of normal intelligence—were receiving thioridazine (50 to 400 mg/day) for one to 4 years. No conclusions can be made as to the function of diagnosis on the basis of this report: The study was retrospective and the 125 patients constituting the sample were diagnostically heterogeneous.

In summary, a great deal of careful and systematic research needs to be done in order to determine the effect of neuroleptics on cognition and learning in children—particularly during long-term administration. It remains to be seen whether high-potency neuroleptics differ from low-potency neuroleptics in their effects in this respect. However, it seems to be safe to conclude that the lowest effective dose of any neuroleptic should be prescribed to youngsters when such a drug is clinically indicated.

IMMEDIATE AND LONG-TERM UNTOWARD EFFECTS

Immediate Untoward Effects

Behavioral toxicity is usually one of the earliest and most common manifestations of excess dose in children, particularly in the young age group. In order to detect behavioral toxicity, a stable behavioral assessment is needed in each child. Behavioral toxicity may be manifested in the form of worsening of preexisting symptoms, or as symptoms de novo: hyperactivity, hypoactivity, irritability, apathy, decrease of verbal production, daze-like behavior, stereotypies, tics, hallucinations, and so on. Administration of haloperidol was reported to be associated with dysphoria and school phobia in children diagnosed as having Tourette's disorder (Mikkelsen et al., 1981).

Extrapyramidal side effects include acute dystonic reactions, parkinsonian untoward effects, and akathisia. Acute dystonic reactions may develop after the first dose of neuroleptic, a few hours after drug administration if received orally, or sooner, if the drug was given intramuscularly (i.m.). They may take the form of oculogyric crisis, torticollis, dystonia of the tongue, trunk, or possibly the esophagus. Usually they can be avoided by a very low starting dose and slow, gradual increments. Diphenhydramine, in a dose of 25 mg orally or i.m., provides rapid relief. Parkinsonian untoward effects usually appear within the first 3 weeks of treatment, and include tremor, cogwheel rigidity, mask-like face, and drooling. In children, extrapyramidal symptoms are best treated by a reduction of dose rather than administration of anticholinergic agents. Anticholinergic agents can cause cognitive dulling and worsening of psychotic disorganization. Moreover, although inconclusive, there are some data to suggest that anticholinergic agents can lower the concentration of neuroleptic in serum (Rivera-Calimlim et al., 1976). Parkinsonian symptoms are rarely seen in young children at therapeutic doses; they are common in school age children and in adolescents.

Table 2 details the untoward effects rated in 40 autistic children, ages 2.33 to 6.92 years, during haloperidol regulation and above-optimal doses (0.5 to 4.0 mg/day); and while receiving placebo (Anderson et al., 1984). The study was double-blind.

Chlorpromazine has epileptogenic effects (Tarjan et al., 1957) and should not be prescribed to patients with seizure disorders.

Neither height nor weight changed significantly in 76 autistic children who participated in two double-blind and placebo-controlled studies of haloperidol over a period of 14 weeks (Green, Campbell, Wolsky et al., 1984). The children were males and females, ages 2 to 7.5 years. The studies employed a within-subjects design, in which children received haloperidol for 4 or (cumulatively) 8 weeks, in doses ranging from 0.5 to 4.0 mg/day, but in most cases about 1.0 mg/day. Most children gained weight (up to a maximum of 3.2 kg); only one child lost 0.79 kg during a 4-week period while receiving haloperidol. Weights were taken weekly, at fixed times.

Laboratory abnormalities related to neuroleptic administration (e.g., blood dyscrasias, liver damage) are rarely reported in children (for review, see DiMascio et al., 1970; Engelhardt & Polizos, 1978).

Long-Term Untoward Effects

Rapid perioral muscular movements, called rabbit syndrome (Ville-neuve, 1972), represent a late-onset extrapyramidal untoward effect. These movements are reduced or controlled by administration of antiparkinsonian drugs and differ from neuroleptic-induced dyskinesias.

Neuroleptic-induced tardive and withdrawal dyskinesias exist in children and adolescents, in both reversible (Perry et al., 1985) and permanent (Gualtieri, Quade et al., 1984; Paulson et al., 1975) form (for review, see Campbell, Grega et al., 1983). Based on retrospective studies, the prevalence of neuroleptic-induced dyskinesias in this age group ranges from 8% (McAndrew et al., 1972) to 51% (Engelhardt & Polizos, 1978; Polizos & Engelhardt, 1980). In a sample of 95 mentally retarded individuals, many of whom were children and adolescents and received neuroleptics on a long-term basis, 35% had "transient withdrawal phenomena," and one-third had tardive dyskinesia (Gualtieri, Breuning et al., 1982). In a multicenter study of 41 patients, ages 3 to 21 years, 16 were institutionalized and mentally retarded; neuroleptic administration ranged from 1 to 132 months (Gualtieri, Quade et al., 1984); 36 percent of the subjects developed tardive or withdrawal dyskinesias. In the only prospective study, the prevalence was 22 percent (Campbell, Grega et al., 1983; Perry et al., 1985), a figure close to some of the more carefully designed studies in adult psychiatric patients (Kane & Smith, 1982). In the prospective and ongoing study of Campbell and associates (design and methods are described in Campbell, Perry et al., 1983), 58 autistic children, ages 3.6 to 7.8 years, received haloperidol maintenance (Perry et al., 1985). In all but the oldest child, daily doses ranged from 0.5 to 3.0 mg (mean 1.0), or 0.02 to 0.22 mg/kg (mean 0.05; Perry et al., 1985). Four raters evaluated the

TABLE 2 Untoward Effects in 40 Autistic Children During Haloperidol and Placebo Administration

Effect	Dose at Which Effect Occurred (mg/day)[a]			Number of Patients[a]			
	A1	B	A2	A1	B	A2	Total
Haloperidol							
Decreased attention span	0.5	–	–	1	0	0	1
Increased motor activity	3.0–4.0	–	–	1	0	0	1
Increased irritability	0.25 b.i.d.–4.0	0.5–4.0	2.0	5	5	1	11
Insomnia	2.0	0.5–4.0	–	0	1	0	1
Depressive affect	–	1.5	–	0	1	0	1
Excessive sedation	0.25 b.i.d.–4.0	0.5–4.0	0.25 b.i.d.–0.5	14	15	2	31
Decreased motor activity	1.5–3.0	–	–	4	0	0	4
Acute dystonic reaction	1.0–4.0	0.5 b.i.d.–4.0	–	4	6	0	10
Drooling	–	1.0–4.0	–	0	2	0	2
Decreased appetite	–	0.5	0.5	0	1	1	2
Pallor	1.5	0.5–1.0	–	1	2	0	3
Hypotensive reaction	0.5 b.i.d.	–	–	1	0	0	1
Tremor	1.5–4.0	1.0	–	4	1	0	5
Cogwheel rigidity	1.0	1.0	–	1	1	0	2
Unsteady gait, motor retardation	1.0–2.0	–	–	2	0	0	2
Bed-wetting	1.0	–	–	1	0	0	1
Urinating on floor	1.0–4.0	–	–	2	0	0	2
Muteness or decreased verbalization	1.5–3.0	–	–	2	0	0	2
Placebo							
Increased aggressiveness against others	4.0	0.5–4.0	1.0–4.0	2	8	9	19
Increased aggressiveness against self	3.0	0.5 b.i.d.–4.0	0.5 b.i.d.–4.0	1	3	2	6
Increased stereotypy	4.0	0.5–4.0	0.5–4.0	2	7	9	18
Increased psychotic speech	–	3.0–4.0	1.0–4.0	0	1	1	2

Behavior	A1	B	A2	A1	B	A2	Total
Increased irritability	1.5	0.5-4.0	0.5-4.0	1	8	7	16
Increased impulsiveness	–	0.5 b.i.d.-4.0	1.0-4.0	0	4	6	10
Increased hyperactivity	3.0	0.5-4.0	0.5-4.0	1	8	14	23
Increased distractibility	4.0	0.5 b.i.d.-4.0	0.5-4.0	1	5	4	10
Decreased tolerance for frustration	–	1.0-1.5	2.0-4.0	0	2	1	3
Disorganization	–	1.0-4.0	1.0-4.0	0	1	1	2
Decreased attention span	2.0-4.0	0.5 b.i.d.-4.0	0.5-4.0	2	8	10	20
Excitement/agitation	4.0	0.5 b.i.d.-4.0	1.0-4.0	2	3	2	7
Increased fidgetiness	3.0-4.0	1.0-4.0	4.0	2	2	1	5
Smearing feces, urinating on floor	4.0	1.0	–	2	1	0	3
Ataxia	–	4.0	–	0	1	0	1
Increased resistance to change	1.0-4.0	–	0.5-4.0	1	0	3	4
Increased negativism	4.0	0.5 b.i.d.-4.0	1.0-4.0	1	2	2	5
Wakefulness at nap time	–	2.0-4.0	1.0-4.0	0	2	3	5
Increased clumsiness	–	3.0	3.0-4.0	0	1	1	2
Aimless wandering	–	2.0	–	0	1	0	1
Decreased verbalization	–	0.5 b.i.d.-4.0	1.0-4.0	0	2	1	3
Decreased exploration of environment	–	–	3.0-4.0	0	0	2	2
Decreased motor activity	2.0	–	1.0	1	0	1	2
Depressive affect	–	–	3.0-4.0	0	0	1	1
Increased withdrawal	–	1.5-4.0	1.0-4.0	0	3	4	7
Decreased appetite	4.0	–	4.0	1	0	2	3
Drooling	4.0	–	–	1	0	0	1
Excessive sedation	1.5	4.0	–	1	1	0	2

SOURCE: Anderson et al., 1984; Reproduced with permission *American Journal of Psychiatry*.

a. A1 = first treatment condition (haloperidol or placebo), B = second treatment condition (placebo or haloperidol), A2 = repetition of first treatment condition.

children independently, following a research protocol, on the Abnormal Involuntary Movements Scale (AIMS; Guy, 1976), on the abridged Simpson Scale (Simpson et al., 1979), on a Timed Stereotypies Rating Scale, and on the CPRS and CGI. The patients were videotaped. Of the 58 children, 13 developed mild to moderately severe neuroleptic-related movements after 3.5 and up to 42.5 months of cumulative drug administration. In four patients the movements developed while on drug, whereas they developed in nine on placebo. In 11 children the movements were de novo, and in 2 an increase in frequency and severity of preexisting movements (stereotypies) was rated; two children developed both types of movements. Clinical diagnosis of neuroleptic-related dyskinesia nearly perfectly agreed with the research diagnostic criteria of Schooler and Kane (1982) as rated on the AIMS. The AIMS items were more reliable than the symptoms on the abridged Simpson Scale. Factor analysis (N = 24) revealed three independent factors: neuroleptic-related dyskinesias, stereotypies, and severity of psychopathology which included stereotypies. For each factor there was a high intermethod and interrater agreement. Within instrument, there was a low correlation between stereotypies and dyskinesias and between severity of psychopathology and stereotypies or dyskinesias. The ratings of videotapes (N = 24) and live ratings showed only minimal differences. The distribution of movements in the 13 patients was as follows: buccal area (N = 10), tongue (N = 4), upper extremities (N = 4), lower extremities (N = 2), trunk (N = 2). One child developed movements in the area of neck, shoulder, and hip; another child had laryngeal and diaphragmatic involvement and emitted throaty sounds. This topography is almost identical to that reported by Gualtieri, Quade et al. (1984), though the psychiatric diagnoses were not specified in that study. Both of these studies are in disagreement with the findings of Engelhardt and Polizos (1978) and Polizos and Engelhardt (1980), who suggest that in children—unlike adults—choreoathetoid movements of upper extremities are seen most frequently. In the Perry et al. (1985) study, dyskinetic movements lasted from 16 days and up to 9 months; in most cases they ceased spontaneously while receiving placebo or no drug at all. Continuous or discontinuous administration of haloperidol had no effect on the development of drug-related movements; nor did sex, even though 4 of the 13 patients who developed movements were females (there were only 11 females in the entire sample). In contrast, Gualtieri, Quade et al. (1984) report that females receiving higher doses of neuroleptics tended to develop neuroleptic-related problems. Drug holidays had no effect in either study. Abrupt or gradual drug withdrawal does not seem to influence the development of dyskinesias (Gualtieri, Quade et al., 1984; Polizos et al., 1973). There is no agreement in the literature as to whether specific neuroleptics present an increased risk (for review, see Campbell, Grega et al., 1983). Tourette-like vocal and motor tics were reported in a few cases in association with chronic neuroleptic treatment (Klawans et al., 1982; Stahl, 1980).

Because many children and adolescents who receive neuroleptics are autistic or mentally retarded, and therefore may exhibit a high rate of abnormal movements (stereotypies) on baseline—prior to neuroleptic administration—it is important to differentiate stereotypies from neuroleptic-induced dyskinesias in these populations. Several issues are involved here (Meiselas et al., 1984). First, some stereotypies and mannerisms, involving the mouth, lips, jaw, or tongue (including the bon-bon sign) are seen in young autistic children who never received pharmacotherapy. They may resemble or be indistinguishable from neuroleptic-related dyskinesias with the same topography. Second, it has been demonstrated that stereotypies can be reduced or controlled by neuroleptics (Anderson et al., 1984; Campbell, Anderson et al., 1978; Cohen et al., 1980) and can reemerge within a week, when the neuroleptic is withdrawn (Campbell, Grega et al., 1983, p. 212; Campbell, Perry et al., 1983). Thus, it may be difficult or impossible to differentiate the withdrawal-dyskinetic movements from reemerging stereotypies that were suppressed by drug. Third, it was demonstrated that a variety of movements, including jaw movements and lip puckering—which occur in preschool age autistic children—are also rated in a large sample of normal controls (N = 101) matched for chronological age and other pertinent variables (Campbell, Grega et al., 1983, p. 213; Cohen et al., 1980). However, the differences between these movements in the two populations were significantly different, both qualitatively and quantitatively. Finally, there are difficulties in examining young and/or severely disturbed and retarded children on scales developed for the measurement of dyskinesias. It is important to ensure that the subject does not have loose baby teeth, cavities, chewing gum, or candy in his or her mouth when examined and/or videotaped for abnormal movements.

In view of these problems each child should be carefully examined and rated on the AIMS or other appropriate scale prior to prescribing a neuroleptic. Careful monitoring at fixed intervals should also be done.

The long-term effects of neuroleptic administration on height and weight were assessed in 42 autistic children in a prospective fashion (Green, Campbell, Wolsky et al., 1984). The design and methods of this study are described elsewhere (Campbell, Perry et al., 1983). The 42 children were 2.0 to 7.6 years of age at the time of enrollment in the study and were receiving haloperidol in daily doses of 0.5 to 3.0 mg. At 6 months of drug maintenance, there was a 4.7-point decrement in mean height percentile, using the growth charts of the National Center of Health Statistics (NCHS; Hamill et al., 1976); this was not statistically significant. At the same time, there was an 8.2-point increase in mean weight percentile ($p < 0.05$). These age-percentile means for height and weight following the 6 month haloperidol maintenance were nearly predictable from height and weight at the time of placement on haloperidol and were not significantly related to dosage, continuous versus intermittent drug administration, sex, or age (Green, Campbell, Wolsky et al., 1984).

Rebound phenomena marked by behavioral deterioration are observed following drug withdrawal, and usually cease spontaneously within a week. They occur even after short-term neuroleptic administration.

Withdrawal symptoms, such as anorexia, nausea, vomiting, diarrhea, weight loss, and diaphoresis were reported upon withdrawal of long-term neuroleptic administration: 5 of 41 patients (12 percent) exhibited some of these symptoms (Gualtieri, Quade et al., 1984).

In a prospective study, designed to assess the long-term efficacy and safety of haloperidol in a diagnostically homogeneous sample of children diagnosed as infantile autism, haloperidol was abruptly withdrawn after 6 months of maintenance and replaced by placebo for a period of 4 weeks (the design and method are described in Campbell, Perry et al., 1983). During the 6 month haloperidol administration, weights were taken monthly, and during the placebo period they were measured weekly at fixed times. In a sample of 20 children, 11 gained weight, 7 showed no change, and 2 lost weight during the 4-week placebo period (Green, Campbell, Wolsky et al., 1984). Maximum weight gain was 0.68 kg in the heaviest subject; maximum loss was 0.80 kg.

Withdrawal related acute behavioral deterioration or neuroleptic-induced supersensitivity psychosis (Chouinard & Jones, 1980) were also reported in this age group. These behavioral symptoms—similar to the above physical withdrawal symptoms—develop upon withdrawal of long-term neuroleptic maintenance; they are qualitatively different from the target symptoms for which the drug was prescribed and usually cease spontaneously. Of 58 autistic children, 1 developed this syndrome one week after withdrawal of haloperidol (3 mg/ day, 0.18 mg/ kg/ day); insomnia, agitation, irritability, hyperactivity, and severe aggressiveness directed against self and others were observed and associated with numerous dyskinetic movements (Campbell, Grega et al., 1983). Both behavioral symptoms and drug-related movements ceased spontaneously within 16 days. Gualtieri, Golden et al. (1984) report that 4 of 41 subjects (less than 10 percent) developed neuroleptic-withdrawal-induced acute behavioral deterioration that ceased spontaneously within 8 weeks, as did the above described physical withdrawal symptoms.

3

STIMULANTS ✓

INDICATIONS

Stimulant medications—mainly methylphenidate, dextroamphetamine, and pemoline—are the drugs of choice in treating children who meet DSM-III (American Psychiatric Association, 1980) criteria for Attention Deficit Disorder with Hyperactivity (ADDH). In the older literature these children were usually described as suffering from hyperkinetic syndrome, minimal brain dysfunction (MBD), or hyperactivity.

In carefully designed, double-blind, placebo-controlled studies, the superiority of the stimulants over placebo in decreasing the cardinal symptoms of ADDH (developmentally inappropriate inattention, impulsivity, and hyperactivity) has been shown consistently.

The prevalence of this disorder in school-aged boys has been variously estimated at up to 20 percent and is severe in about 5 percent of them (Wender, 1971). The prevalence is less in girls. Stimulant medications are the most commonly prescribed drugs during childhood. Sprague and Sleator (1977) reported that over 500,000 children in the United States were treated with methylphenidate.

CONTRAINDICATIONS

The stimulants have been found to exacerbate symptoms in pervasive developmental disorder (infantile autism), schizophrenic disorder, and borderline personality disorder. In children with these conditions, the stimulants increase psychotic disorganization, exacerbate pre-existing stereotypies and precipitate stereotypies and tics de novo. Furthermore, in vulnerable children, development of Tourette's disorder may be hastened (Lowe et al., 1982).

TABLE 3   Representative Simulants, Doses, and Age Restrictions in Children and Adolescents

Generic Name (Trade Name)	Dosage		Age Restrictions
Methylphenidate	Range	10 to 60 mg/day	6 years or older
(Ritalin)	Average	20 to 30 mg/day	
Dextroamphetamine sulfate (Dexedrine)	Range	2.5 to 40 mg/day	3 years or older
Magnesium pemoline (Cylert)	Range	37.5 to 112.5 mg/day	6 years or older

DOSAGE

Table 3 gives the currently recommended doses of stimulants for use in children. At the present time, methylphenidate is the most widely prescribed of the stimulants and will be considered the prototype in reviewing issues regarding dosage.

Prior to drug administration, a baseline of target behaviors in the home and school environments should be obtained.

Most clinicians feel that the drug should be individually titrated. Dosage initiation should begin with a small, perhaps ineffective dose and should be gradually increased until the desired clinical effect is achieved, clinical improvement reaches a plateau, untoward effects prevent further increase, or maximum allowable dosage is reached.

Peak blood levels of methylphenidate are attained from 1 to 2½ hours after oral administration (Gualtieri, Wafgin et al., 1982; Shaywitz et al., 1982). Once therapeutic dosages are reached, one may see an amelioration of target symptoms within 30 minutes to 1 hour.

Pharmacokinetic data have shown a 2.5-hour half-life for methylphenidate (Winsberg et al., 1982). This is consistent with the 4 to 6 hour duration of clinical effects and it is the rationale for prescribing the medication at approximate dosage times of 8:00 a.m. and noon. Methylphenidate is now available in a sustained release 20-mg tablet with an approximate duration of action of 8 hours. This formulation appears to be useful for some children. In one study, children whose peak serum methylphenidate levels were below 7 ng/ml failed to show any behavioral effect (Shaywitz et al., 1982).

Sprague and Werry (1973) and Sprague and Sleator (1973) found that 0.3 mg/kg of methylphenidate produced the greatest increment in short-term memory tasks in the laboratory and, at the same time, statistically significant improvement on teacher and physician ratings. It must be remembered that these results were obtained in the laboratory and, clinically, it has been found that higher doses may be necessary. A reasonable maximum clinical dose range is from 0.5 to 0.7 mg/kg. At higher doses, increasingly severe side effects emerge. At 1.0 mg/kg, 20 percent to 50 percent of children display severe side effects: gastrointestinal symptoms, anorexia, weight loss, insomnia, and worsening of behavior (Sprague & Werry, 1973; Winsberg et al., 1982).

The pharmacokinetics of magnesium pemoline differ significantly from the other stimulants; its serum half-life is about 12 hours, which permits once-daily dosage, making a noon-time dose in school unnecessary. Starting dosage is 37.5 mg/day with weekly increments of 18.75 mg. The usual effective dose range is 56.25 mg to 75 mg daily with a maximum recommended dose of 112 mg/day. Significant clinical benefit may not be evident using the recommended dosage schedule until the third or fourth week or longer.

DRUG HOLIDAYS AND PERIODIC REASSESSMENT WITHOUT MEDICATION

The symptomatology of ADDH children often varies according to the specific environment. Often during weekends, vacations, summertime, and periods of lower stress, these children may function adequately without medication. Sometimes, with maturation, it is possible to stop the medication permanently and maintain gains. Periodic assessments without medication are indicated.

Sleator et al. (1974) followed 42 hyperactive children treated with methylphenidate for 1 to 2 years. Eleven (26 percent) of these children continued to function adequately in school both behaviorally and academically without medication following a one-month placebo period. Only 40 percent showed worsening on placebo. Gittelman-Klein, Katz et al. (1976) found that 5 percent of hyperactive children maintained their gains when methylphenidate was discontinued after three months.

SHORT- AND LONG-TERM EFFICACY

Effect on Behavioral Symptoms

Rapoport, Buchsbaum et al. (1978) administered a single acute dose of 0.5 mg/kg (mean dose 15.80 ± 3.90 mg) of dextroamphetamine or placebo to 14 normal prepubertal boys (mean age 10.10 ± 2.10 years) in a double-blind crossover study. They had mean IQs of 131.0 ± 18.0. None had previously taken amphetamines. These boys with no abnormal behavioral or learning difficulties reacted to stimulant administration in much the same way as children with MBD or hyperkinesis. They showed decreased motor activity (decreased actometer counts, low voice, and hypoactivity in the interview), generally improved attentional performance (faster reaction time, superior memory, and improved vigilance), and decreased galvanic skin response amplitude. After drug administration, these normal children appeared unusually inactive. Mood effects were not significant except that some children said, "I feel funny, not like myself." A marked behavioral rebound occurred about 5 hours after dextroamphetamine but not after placebo. This rebound consisted of excitability and talkativeness. In addition, 10 experienced overactivity, 9 had insomnia, and 3 had stomach aches and mild nausea. During the rebound period 3 also experienced euphoria. The authors' major conclusions were (1) that MBD children probably do not have a paradoxical response to stimulant medication; (2) hypotheses of dopamine depletion or low arousal are not necessary to explain the reaction of MBD children to stimulants; (3) no diagnostic significance should be inferred from good response to stimulants; (4) late afternoon behavioral difficulties in medicated children may be related to drug action (rebound) and not simply to wearing off of the therapeutic effect; and (5) because the rebound behavior of normals resembled clinical hyperactivity, the authors suggested that altered receptor sensitivity in MBD children should be investigated.

Rapoport, Buchsbaum et al. (1980) published additional data on these 14 normal prepubertal boys and compared them to hyperactive boys and normal college aged men under the same experimental conditions. The 15 hyperactive boys (mean age 9.44 ± 2.12 years) had mean IQs of 112 ± 18; 10 had been previously treated with stimulants and were "good responders," whereas 5 had not received stimulants before. Mean dose of dextroamphetamine was 16.17 ± 4.60 mg.

The college aged men consisted of two groups (age range between 18 and 30). The "high dose" group had a mean age 22.50 ± 2.80, with a mean IQ of 122.50 ± 9.60, and received a mean dose of dextroamphetamine of 0.45 ± 0.04 mg/kg. The "low dose" group had a mean age of 22.20 ± 3.17 and a mean IQ of 125.70 ± 5.92. They received a mean dose of dextroamphetamine of 0.23 ± 0.02 mg/kg. Of the 31 men, 13 had no prior experience with stimulant medication. None had a history of childhood learning or behavior problems.

All subjects knew the identity of the test drug. The subjects were evaluated over three sessions: a baseline session and two experimental sessions in which they were given a single dose of placebo or dextroamphetamine in a random, double-blind design.

Truncal motor activity was measured for two hours beginning a half hour after drug was given. The normal boys (p < .002), the hyperactive boys (p < .0001) and the low-dose men (p < .03) all showed significant decreases from baseline when given dextroamphetamine. There was no difference in the high-dose men between baseline and dextroamphetamine. The hyperactive boys showed a mean decrease of 44 percent in activity counts on dextroamphetamine compared with level on placebo. This was significantly different from the other three groups that showed mean decreases of 24 percent in normal boys and 9 percent in low-dose men, and a mean increase of 3 percent in high-dose men. On self-reported mood, both groups of boys reported they "felt funny," and the hyperactive boys also noted increase in being "tired." Both groups of men reported increased euphoria, more energy, and feeling more talkative.

Behavioral ratings by blind interviewers on the Children's Psychiatric Rating Scale (CPRS) noted increased hypoactivity in the normal boys, decreased restlessness in the hyperactive boys, increased activity and euphoria in the high-dose men, and no change in the low-dose men. Vigilance as measured by Rosvold's Continuous Performance Test was increased significantly in both groups of boys and in the high dose men. Memory for a verbal learning task increased significantly in all four groups. Reaction time decreased in all groups except the high-dose men. All groups tended to increase their total verbal output.

The authors noted that all four groups showed decreased motor activity and enhanced memory on dextroamphetamine, although this did not always attain statistical significance. Both the normal and hyperactive boys showed improved vigilance and reaction time. Thus the data do not support any differences in the effects of dextroamphetamine between normal and hyperactive children. Clearly, response or nonresponse to dextroamphetamine cannot be used as a diagnostic confirmation.

The most marked difference between children and adults was the effect of dextroamphetamine on mood. Increased euphoria, decreased tiredness, and increased energy levels were significant only in adults. One can speculate that this may be partially responsible for the finding that treatment of children with stimulants for hyperactivity has not been reported to increase later abuse (Weiss et al., 1979).

In a classic paper, Bradley (1937) reported staff observations of the behavioral responses of a heterogeneous group of 30 children in a residential facility (21 boys and 9 girls; ages 5 to 14 years) to single morning doses of racemic amphetamine sulfate (dose range 10 to 30 mg; modal dose 20 mg) over the course of one week. The children were of normal intelligence and their behavior disorders "were of sufficient severity to warrant hospitalization." The range of primary diagnoses included "specific educational disabilities," "retiring schizoid child," and "aggressive, egocentric epileptic child," among others. A dramatic improvement of school performance was observed in 14 of the 30 children. These children displayed increased interest in school material, a "drive" to accomplish and complete their tasks, quicker comprehension, and more accurate performance. Effects were evident on the first day of administration and persisted up until the day of withdrawal. In terms of affective behaviors, 15 children became "distinctly subdued in their emotional responses." Clinically, this change was felt to reflect a greater ability to modulate the severity and range of affective responses and was viewed as a positive treatment outcome. The subdued behavior was associated with an improved sense of well-being and greater interest in the surroundings. The improved school performance was not a direct consequence of amphetamine's positive effect on modulation of emotional behavior because there were mutually exclusive subgroups of children who responded with either improved school performance or more subdued behavior. Only seven children displayed *both* improved school performance and subdued behavior.

The effect of dextroamphetamine on the school performance and behavior of a heterogeneous sample of 52 fifth and sixth grade children (34 boys and 18 girls; mean age 11.6 ± 1.08 [SD] years) was examined in a double-blind, placebo-controlled crossover study (Conners et al., 1967). The dextrorotatory isomer was selected for this study because of its greater potency in the elicitation of central excitatory effects than the racemic mixture (benzedrine). The children were referred by two inner-city public elementary schools. Many of the children were referred primarily because of problem behaviors such as defiance, aggressiveness, impulsiveness, inattention, and restlessness. Others were referred because of poor academic performance, for example, poor reading skills. The subjects were randomly assigned to one of two orders of drug condition: dextroamphetamine-placebo or placebo-dextroamphetamine. Each treatment condition lasted one month; the crossover occurred on the day after the first month of treatment. A fixed 10-mg dose of dextroamphetamine sulfate or matching placebo was administered in the morning. Teachers and children were blind to the nature of the medication condition, On baseline and at the end of each treatment condition, teachers employed a symptom checklist to rate the children in three broad areas: classroom behavior, group participation, and attitude toward authority. In addition, teachers provided written global impressions of changes during each month of treatment. The children also were tested to measure intellectual ability ("Factor I") and assertiveness and drive ("Factor II"). The authors hoped to determine whether dextroamphetamine's positive effects on school performance and behavior were due to an improvement of intellectual functioning or an epiphenomenon of increased motivation. Dextroamphetamine was significantly superior to placebo in reducing the severity of items in all three areas of behavior on the teacher rating scale. In terms of the teachers' global ratings, the majority of children showed significant worsening when switched from drug to placebo and significant improvement when switched from placebo to drug. Dextroamphetamine was significantly superior to placebo in increasing objective test scores related to "energetic, decisive, and quick response, combining an expansive and self-assertive quality with a fast speed and tempo." The significant increases of Factor II scores and lack of any significant dextroamphetamine effect on scores related to intellectual function (Factor I) were interpreted to mean that observed improvement of school performance was a result of positive changes in motivation. The children in this study were from economically and psychosocially disadvantaged backgrounds. These factors are quite likely to have influenced the development and severity of many of the target symptoms. Therefore, the salutary effects of dextroamphetamine in this sample could indicate that the drug's effectiveness is not necessarily dependent on the presence of an underlying (subtle) organic disturbance. Rather, the drug's effectiveness could be related to a primary effect on motivation.

Dextroamphetamine's ability to influence motor activity levels was studied in a sample of 42 learning disabled children (Conners et al., 1969). These children were randomly assigned to a four-week outpatient trial of dextroamphetamine or placebo. Dosage was initiated with 10 mg/day in divided doses and, in most children, increased to 25 mg/day by the final week of treatment. Parents recorded weekly activity in different situations (e.g., dinner table, watching television and shopping) on a special scale and completed a symptom rating scale. The parent ratings showed a significant reduction of hyperkinetic symptoms in children treated with dextroamphetamine. Weekly activity levels were negatively related to dosage increments of dextroamphetamine.

In the pharmacological management of hyperactive and learning disabled children, it is desirable to have a choice of alternative drugs that can be tried on an empirical basis. A controlled trial compared magnesium pemoline with dextroamphetamine and placebo in the outpatient treatment of 81 hyperactive children (ages 6 to 12 years; mean 8.24 years) of normal intelligence with poor attention span, disruptive behavior, and poor academic performance (Conners et al., 1972). Children were randomly assigned to one of three eight-week treatment conditions: magnesium pemoline, dextroamphetamine sulfate, or placebo; each testing condition contained 27 subjects. Magnesium pemoline and dextroamphetamine were initiated with morning dosages of 25 mg and 5 mg, respectively; increments occurred according to a fixed schedule with maximal dosages of magnesium pemoline (125 mg) and dextroamphetamine (40 mg) attained at the beginning of the fifth week. The emergence of side effects was the limiting factor in the upward adjustment of dose. The optimal dosages of magnesium pemoline and dextroamphetamine ranged from 25 to 125 mg/day (mean 82 mg) and 5 to 40 mg/day (mean 20 mg), respectively. On baseline and at the end of weeks four and and eight of treatment, rating scales were completed by teachers (39 items) and parents (93 items). Subscale scores based on factor analysis of the items were computed for each child. In addition, teachers and parents completed an abbreviated ten-item scale on baseline and at intervals of two weeks, and provided global ratings of improvement at weeks four and eight of treatment. Globally, teachers and physicians concurred that both drugs were significantly superior to placebo at the end of the fourth and eighth weeks.

On these global ratings, a greater percentage of the children receiving dextroamphetamine was rated as "much improved" as compared with children receiving magnesium pemoline. On the teacher rating scale, both drugs were superior to placebo in reducing factor scores pertaining to defiance, inattention, and hyperactivity at the end of eight weeks; the significant positive effects of dextroamphetamine appeared sooner and were evident at the end of four weeks. At the end of eight weeks, dextroamphetamine was superior to placebo in reducing parent rated scores for the following factors: conduct, impulsivity, immaturity, antisocial, and hyperactivity; whereas, magnesium pemoline positively influenced factor scores related to conduct, impulsivity, and antisocial. No significant differences were detected between the drugs on any of the teacher or parent factor scores at the end of eight weeks. The onset of dextroamphetamine's therapeutic effect occurred more quickly than that of magnesium pemoline; however, few, if any, important differences between the two drugs could be detected at the end of eight weeks (Conners et al., 1972).

In addition to providing an alternative drug, pemoline's longer duration of action and the ease of once a day administration obviate difficulties associated with drug administration during school hours (Conners & Taylor, 1980). In order to explore the efficacy and safety of pemoline further, it was compared to placebo and to methylphenidate, the most widely used stimulant, in an eight-week trial involving 60 hyperactive children (57 boys and 3 girls; ages 6 years to 11 years, 1 month; Conners & Taylor, 1980). The children were pervasively hyperactive—both at home and school—of normal intelligence and from stable family situations. They were randomly assigned to one of three eight-week outpatient treatment regimens: pemoline, methylphenidate, or placebo. Pemoline and methylphenidate were initiated at dosages of 37.5 mg/day and 10 mg/day, respectively. Increments were made on a weekly basis until maximum dosages of pemoline (112.5 mg/day) and methylphenidate (60 mg/day) were achieved or until limiting side effects emerged. The final mean dosages of pemoline and methylphenidate were 60 mg/day (2.25 mg/kg/day) and 22.0 mg/day (0.82 mg/kg/day), respectively. The previously described 93-item (parent) and 39-item (teacher) rating scales were administered on baseline and after weeks four and eight of treatment. In addition, parents and teachers completed an abbreviated 10-item scale, which consisted of items common to both longer instruments, on a weekly basis. The treating physicians, parents, and teachers also provided their global impressions of change over the course of treatment. Both drugs positively influenced factor scores associated with impulsivity; the onset of pemoline's positive effect on the impulsivity factor score was more gradual. Both drugs were significantly superior to placebo in terms of reducing the parents' severity ratings on the abbreviated questionnaire containing 10 items related to the hyperkinetic syndrome. Parents rated the children two weeks after drug discontinuation (week ten) with the 10-item questionnaire. On this instrument, children receiving methylphenidate showed a rapid return to baseline levels of symptom severity following discontinuation, whereas children who received pemoline appeared better able to maintain their positive gains. At the end of weeks four and eight, parents' global impressions indicated that both drugs significantly reduced the seriousness of their child's problem. Teacher ratings also showed the drugs to be effective in the reduction of "defiance" and "hyperactivity" factor scores. The reductions of these scores relative to placebo were more pronounced at week four and teachers were more impressed with the efficacy of methylphenidate as compared to pemoline. A possible explanation for the teachers' impression of methylphenidate's superiority over pemoline is that methylphenidate may have a quicker onset of action. Thus the therapeutic action of methylphenidate may be more apparent than that of pemoline in the earlier part of the school day. The global impressions of staff were that both drugs were significantly superior to placebo and did not differ from each other.

The symptomatologic overlap between mental retardation and attention deficit disorder with hyperactivity (ADDH), and the salutary effects of stimulants in the latter condition prompted clinical trials of these medications in mentally retarded children. The therapeutic efficacy of amphetamine was compared with thioridazine and placebo in a six-month trial, under double-blind conditions, in a sample of 21 hospitalized mentally retarded children (14 boys and 7 girls; ages 7 to 12 years) who manifested persisting hyperactivity for at least one year (Alexandris & Lundell, 1968). The IQ range of the sample was between 55 and 85. Children were randomly assigned to one of three treatment conditions: amphetamine (n = 6), thioridazine (n = 7), or placebo (n = 8). Mean daily amphetamine and thioridazine dosages at the termination of the study were 52 mg (range 7.5 to 75 mg) and 95 mg (range 30 to 150 mg), respectively. For each individual, dosage increments were made on a weekly basis until maximal therapeutic responses were observed; the emergence of "mild side effects such as weight loss or gain, impaired sleep or appetite" did not limit upward adjustment of dose. Ratings of symptom severity were conducted weekly by individual staff members using a 14-item evaluation form. A "final improvement rating" was derived from these forms at the conclusion of the study. Thioridazine was superior to placebo in improving scores in most areas (including hyperkinesis, concentration, attention, aggressiveness, sociability, interpersonal relationship, comprehension, mood, work interest and capacity, and class standing). Only scores in academic achievement (i.e., reading, spelling, and arithmetic) failed to improve. Amphetamine was superior to placebo in only two areas: comprehension and work interest.

Although the sample sizes were small and, therefore, conclusions must be viewed as tentative, thioridazine was superior to amphetamine in this sample of hyperactive mentally retarded children.

The short-term efficacy of methylphenidate in the treatment of inattention, impulsivity, and hyperactivity was studied in a sample of ten mentally retarded children (seven boys and three girls; ages 4.58 to 15 years; IQ range from 49 to 77; Varley & Trupin, 1982). These children were living at home and attending special education programs. The study was double-blind and placebo-controlled and lasted for 21 days. Children were randomly assigned to a sequence of three drug conditions: two dosage levels of methylphenidate (usually 0.3 and 0.6 mg/kg/day) and placebo. The impressions of teachers and parents were obtained daily and reflected in scores on the ten-item Conners abbreviated questionnaire. Five children responded positively to medication, with teacher and parent scores showing significant improvement under the high dose condition ($p < .05$ and $< .02$, respectively). Significant improvement was not shown for the low dose condition. In general, the response rate of this small retarded sample was lower, and the children were less sensitive to the positive effects of methylphenidate than were ADDH children with normal intelligence.

Aman (1984) concluded that stimulant drugs were less effective in mentally retarded samples than in children of normal intelligence with ADDH. He speculated that the drugs may further narrow and constrict attention in many retarded patients with a severe preexisting "narrow focus of attention."

The relative merits of methylphenidate alone, behavior therapy alone, and the combination of the two interventions in the treatment of attention deficit disorder with hyperactivity were studied in a sample of 34 pervasively hyperactive children of normal intelligence (32 boys and 2 girls; mean age 8 years, 2 months) (Gittelman-Klein, Klein, Abikoff et al., 1976). Although stimulant medications are extremely effective for the short-term management of inattention and hyperkinesis, concern over adverse long-term side effects, especially on growth, stimulated interest in the presumably "less toxic" behavioral interventions. The children accepted into this study were between the ages of 6 and 12 years, of normal intelligence, and displayed evidence of hyperactivity and behavior problems at home and in school, as reflected in elevated factor scores on the Conners Teacher Rating Scale and confirmed by the actual observations of trained personnel in the classrooms. In their classrooms hyperactive children and normal classmates were observed for 16-

minute periods during structured lessons and rated in five categories: (1) interference (disruption of classroom work); (2) off-task (not attending to lesson); (3) gross motor movement (out-of-seat activity); (4) minor motor movement (fidgetiness); and (5) solicitation (seeking the teacher's attention). The Conners Teacher Rating Scale, formal classroom observations, and global impressions of improvement by teachers, parents, and physicians served as the outcome measures at the end of the eight-week treatment period. The ADDH children were randomly assigned to one of three treatment conditions: behavior therapy with methylphenidate (n = 13); methylphenidate (n = 12); or behavior therapy with placebo (n = 9). Methylphenidate dosage was initiated with 10 mg/day, in two divided doses, and increments were made weekly to a maximum of 80 mg/day. Dosage increments were made only if "problematic behavior" persisted during the preceding week. At the end of eight weeks, dosage ranged from 10 to 60 mg/day (mean 35.6 mg/day). Behavior therapy was administered by teachers and parents according to operant conditioning principles. Teachers provided tokens for a variety of positive behaviors: "Listening to teachers, no calling out, not interrupting, not leaving seat, doing the work, and not disturbing other children." Parents positively reinforced compliance with such rules as cooperating, and not fighting with siblings.

When compared with children receiving behavior therapy alone, the children receiving methylphenidate, either alone or with behavior therapy, showed significantly lower factor scores related to Conduct Disorder, Inattention, Hyperactivity, and Sociability on the Teacher Rating Scale. There were no significant differences on these scores between children receiving methylphenidate alone and methylphenidate with behavior therapy. At the end of the eight-week treatment period, comparisons of normal children with the hyperactive children in each of the three conditions were made using the Conners Teacher Rating Scale. These scores for hyperactive children receiving the combined therapy of methylphenidate and behavior therapy were indistinguishable from those for normals on the factors of Conduct Disorder, Inattention, and Hyperactivity. The scores for children receiving methylphenidate alone resembled those for normals on the factors of Conduct Disorder and Hyperactivity. The posttreatment Teacher Rating Scale scores for hyperactive children receiving only behavior therapy remained significantly worse than those of normals.

In terms of classroom observations, all hyperactive children receiving methylphenidate, with or without behavior therapy, were significantly less disruptive than those receiving behavior therapy alone. Moreover, children receiving the combined treatment of methylphenidate and behavior therapy were indistinguishable from their normal classmates. Global improvement ratings by teachers and physicians favored the children receiving medication; and there was also the suggestion in their ratings that the combined treatment was superior to medication alone. Globally, mothers rated the children in all three active treatment groups as improved. On the mothers' global ratings of improvement, no statistically significant differences between conditions were detected.

In general, medication proved to be a superior intervention to the administration of behavior therapy in the eight-week trial. Moreover, if one considers the cost-effectiveness of medication, (compared to that of behavior therapy, which requires time and energy of high-level, trained personnel), the superiority and feasibility of medication in the treatment of this highly prevalent disorder becomes even more apparent. It should be emphasized that medication proved effective in a sample of children selected because of relatively severe disruptiveness. Moreover, in this sample, medication was superior to behavior therapy even though the latter was of an intensive nature—administered both in school and at home. The data dispute claims that behavior therapy is equally effective or superior to medication, although the results do suggest that a comprehensive program of behavior therapy may provide additional benefits in a regimen of medication.

D-Amphetamine (Campbell, Fish, & David, 1972; Campbell, Fish, Korein et al., 1972) and L-amphetamine (Campbell et al., 1976) had only small positive effects, if any, in autistic children. These effects, consisting mainly of decreased hyperactivity, were outweighed by untoward effects, particularly stereotypies de novo, worsening of preexisting stereotypies, withdrawal and irritability, aggressiveness, psychosis, and excessive sedation. Only single case reports describe beneficial effects of methylphenidate in the autistic child (Geller et al., 1981).

Effect on Cognition

The monthly school records of 19 children (14 boys and 5 girls, ages 9 to 14 years) of normal intelligence (IQ range 78 to 144) treated with racemic amphetamine sulfate (dosage range 10 to 30 mg; model dose 20 mg) were reviewed (Bradley & Bowen, 1940). These children were residents of a long-term psychiatric facility and their general school adjustment showed improvement with amphetamine. Diagnostically, they formed a heterogeneous group of behavior disordered children: schizoid personality (n = 5), convulsive disorder (n = 4), specific reading disability (n = 3) and a miscellaneous group of behavior problems (n = 7). Two monthly school records were compared for each child, namely a medication-free month and a month during which amphetamine was administered. Monthly school records were sufficiently detailed to provide meaningful information in three areas: behavior and attitude in the classroom, arithmetic achievement, and spelling achievement. The group was selected for study because of improvement in behavior and attitude while receiving amphetamine. Teacher reports during the month of active medication emphasized the following types of changes: increased attention and concentration, less distractibility, more conscientiousness, greater interest, less daydreaming, and less emotional volatility. The authors wished to determine whether the improvements in behavior and attitude were associated with improved school performance in general, or if some areas of academic functioning were more consistently affected than others. While receiving amphetamines, 17 children increased the number of standard pages completed in their arithmetic texts; moreover, the number of children showing the normal rate of monthly progress in arithmetic rose from 6 to 14. There was great variability in the amount of arithmetic progress shown by individual children. In contrast to the primarily positive effect of amphetamine on arithmetic performance, its effect on monthly spelling progress was mixed; 9 children improved and 10 worsened on this measure. A "dissociation" between arithmetic and spelling performance was seen in 10 children, with improvement in one or the other but not both. Also, in most instances (17 cases), behavior and arithmetic performance changed in the same positive direction, whereas no obvious relationship appeared to exist between behavior and spelling performance. This differential effect of amphetamine most likely reflects differences in the cognitive processes associated with these two scholastic tasks.

The influence of dextroamphetamine on intellectual functions related to poor school performance was examined in a sample of 42 children (30 boys and 12 girls) whose primary complaint was some form of learning disability (Conners et al., 1969). The average age of these children was about ten years. Academic problems as the sole difficulty occurred in about 27 percent of the sample; the remainder had associated behavior problems. After a detailed pretreatment assessment, children were randomly assigned to a four-week outpatient trial of either dextroamphetamine or placebo. Dosage was initiated with 10 mg/day, in two divided doses, and increments were made such that the maximum dose of 25 mg/day was reached by the final week of treatment. The modal dosage received by the majority of children was 25 mg/day; loss of appetite and sleep disruption necessitated dosage reduction in some children. The entire pretreatment assessment battery was repeated at the end of the four weeks. The assessment battery included standardized tests of intellectual functioning, academic achievement and ability, visuo-spatial-motor coordination, and perceptual function.

Dextroamphetamine improved arithmetic performance significantly. Reading performance showed a nonsignificant trend toward improvement in the children receiving dextroamphetamine. Porteus Maze quotients improved in children receiving dextroamphetamine. The completion of these mazes requires planning and reflective thought and, therefore, improved scores do not only imply faster completion but also inhibition of "impulsive darting." Dextroamphetamine improved the ability of children to copy increasingly complex designs and recognize geometric designs embedded in distracting backgrounds. Auditory synthesis, or the ability to connect discrete phonemic components into complete words, was improved by dextroamphetamine. This ability has been shown to be defective in many learning disabled children. Improved auditory synthesis was interpreted to reflect a positive influence on attention in the auditory mode. Dextroamphetamine resulted in improved performance on a paired-associate learning task.

The effects of an eight-week trial of treatment with either magnesium pemoline (maximum dose 125 mg/day) or dextroamphetamine (maximum dose 40 mg/day) on cognitive performance were examined in a heterogeneous group of 81 hyperkinetic children aged 6 to 12 years (Conners et al., 1972). A large battery of formal psychological assessments was obtained on baseline and at the end of the eighth week of treatment. These tests assessed areas of intelligence, visuo-spatial-motor coordination, attention, perceptual function, reading and language abilities, and motor development. On the formal psychological tests, both drugs were shown to improve spelling, reading, Porteus IQs, perceptual abilities, and visuo-motor coordination significantly.

The effect of pemoline on cognitive performance was compared to that of methylphenidate and placebo in an eight-week trial involving 60 hyperactive children (Conners & Taylor, 1980). After dosage regulation, the final mean dosages of pemoline and methylphenidate were 60 mg/day and 22 mg/day, respectively. A large battery of formal psychological tests was administered on baseline and at the end of the eight-week treatment period. Active drug treatment was significantly superior to placebo in improving full-scale and performance IQs, but children receiving either drug did not differ from one another on these measures. There were no significant effects of treatment with either drug on verbal IQ. Pemoline appeared to be superior to placebo in terms of improving scores on the Porteus Maze and Harris-Goodenough Draw-A-Man tests. However, the drug effects on the cognitive functions reflected in these tests were of a modest nature.

Methylphenidate's therapeutic efficacy in terms of improving cognitive performance and academic achievement was examined in a group of 61 children (47 boys and 14 girls; mean age 10.75 years) who presented with a specific developmental disorder of reading but without evidence of cross-situational hyperactivity (Gittelman-Klein & Klein, 1976). The investigators were interested in determining whether methylphenidate has a salutary effect on the school performance of children who did not show evidence of inattention, hyperkinesis, or a primary behavior disorder and were free of significant psychopathology. The major issue addressed in this study was to see if reported improvements in the academic performance of children receiving methylphenidate were due to a primary effect on cognitive processes or secondary to improved behaviors. The 61 children in this study were of normal intelligence (IQ $\geq$ 80) but their reading performance was at least two years below grade level. The majority of the children were from stable, nurturing home environments and had received prior academic remediation. The 61 children were randomly assigned to one of two 12-week outpatient medication conditions: methylphenidate (n = 29) or placebo (n = 32). Dosage was administered so that the best tolerated dose was achieved by the end of 4 weeks (the maximum allowable dose was 60 mg/day). At the end of 12 weeks, the methylphenidate dosage ranged from 20 to 60 mg/day (mean 52 mg/day). The medication was administered in a double-blind fashion. Assessments were performed on baseline and repeated after 4 and 12 weeks of treatment. The assessments included formal tests of intellectual and cognitive performance, academic achievement, visual-motor coordination, learning ability, and attention. Teachers also provided their global impressions of academic performance in reading and arithmetic. Methylphenidate positively influenced performance IQ, Porteus Maze scores, visual sequential memory, visual-motor integration, and other cognitive measures, but the two groups did not differ in their academic achievement at the end of 12 weeks. Neither formal achievement test scores nor teachers' global ratings could distinguish the two groups at 12 weeks. An initial positive drug effect on arithmetic performance was detected at the end of week four but disappeared at the end of the 12-week trial. The data suggest that the administration of methylphenidate for the sole purpose of improving academic achievement in children without other behavioral difficulties, e.g., inattention, impulsivity and/or hyperactivity, is not warranted (Gittelman-Klein & Klein, 1976).

Aman and Werry (1982) compared the effects of diazepam to those of methylphenidate and placebo in 15 outpatients, age 6.83 to 12.08 years (mean 9.61), with IQs of 81 to 135 (mean 104.8) who had severe reading retardation; their reading age was at least 24 months below their mental age. Subjects were randomly assigned in equal numbers to a crossover design in which each subject acted as his or her own control. Each drug was administered for six days with a one day placebo washout period between conditions. Diazepam was given in doses of 0.10 mg/kg; methylphenidate in doses of 0.35 mg/kg. Children were rated on over 20 measurements including manifest anxiety scale, matching familiar figures (MFF), auditory-visual integration (AV), continuous performance test (CPT), seat movement, motor performance (mazes), and standardized reading scores. Most drug-related changes were in areas unrelated to basic cognitive deficits. Both diazepam and methylphenidate caused significant reductions in omission errors in the CPT, suggesting they improved attention span. Both drugs caused nonsignificant improvements in reading behaviors (self-correction rate, error rate, and repetition rate). The slight improvements appeared to result from enhanced performance and not from improved acquisition abilities. The authors concluded that neither drug was useful in treating children with severe specific reading retardation.

The effects of two dosage levels of methylphenidate (0.3 and 0.6 mg/kg) and placebo on tasks reflective of symbolic language processing were examined in nine boys (ages 9 to 15 years; mean 11.71 years) with attention deficit disorder and hyperactivity (Ballinger et al., 1984). The medication trials on each dosage level and placebo lasted for one week and testing was performed one hour after morning administration on the seventh day. The study was conducted double-blind. The children were of normal intelligence but were delayed in their reading levels;

reading levels of six boys were more than two years below the expected level (range 0.5 to 5.5 years). Prior to their enrollment in this study, the children were shown to be "positive responders" to the behavioral effects of methylphenidate in a double-blind crossover study that included placebo. In a dose-dependent fashion, methylphenidate increased the speed of decisions reflecting cognitive processes associated with symbolic language. While receiving methylphenidate, the children were more quickly able to decide whether a sentence was a true description of a diagram and whether two members of a pair of letters were the same or different. The children showing the greatest amount of reading lag benefited the least from methylphenidate on the letter matching task. However, as in previous reports, methylphenidate was without any significant effect on measures derived from a standardized test of oral reading and comprehension. The authors related their results to the possibility of methylphenidate's differential effect on the two symptom clusters of ADDH, such as disinhibition of motor activity and problems with arousal. Complex measures may fail to demonstrate a positive effect of methylphenidate due to its differential influence on these two symptom clusters. For example, a longer response latency could represent a positive effect on impulsivity rather than an impairment of central decision-making processes. The authors concluded that the inclusion of information-processing tasks would provide useful information regarding methylphenidate's positive effects in children with ADDH and learning difficulties.

IMMEDIATE AND LONG-TERM
UNTOWARD EFFECTS

The stimulants are indirect catecholaminergic agonists and many of their side effects are directly attributable to their psychopharmacologic properties. In general, the side effects are due to the peripheral or central effects of these drugs and are often dose related.

Increased sympathetic nervous system tone may result in increased pulse rates, elevations of both diastolic and systolic blood pressures, and weak bronchodilation and respiratory stimulant action. These drugs are also associated with gastrointestinal irritability, including diarrhea, constipation, and dryness of mouth. Nausea, vomiting, anorexia, and weight loss are relatively frequently reported and may be due to central as well as peripheral actions. Central effects include irritability, restlessness, insomnia, alteration of mood (including mood lability), over-stimulation, and precipitation of psychosis. These drugs also affect central involuntary motor centers (e.g., nigrostriatal pathways) resulting in exacerbation or precipitation of motor and phonic tics, dyskinesias, worsening of preexisting stereotypies, and stereotypies de novo.

Tics and Tourette's Disorder

An increased incidence of motor tics has been reported in hyperactive children taking stimulant medication. Denckla et al. (1976) reported 14 (0.92 percent) of 1520 ADDH children developed tic while receiving methylphenidate, and in 6 (0.39 percent) preexisting tics worsened. Following methylphenidate's discontinuation, only 1 of the 14 newly developed tics persisted and all 6 exacerbated tics returned to premedication levels.

Lowe et al. (1982) reported that both dextroamphetamine and methylphenidate precipitated Tourette's disorder in 15 cases (13 males, ages 5 to 11 years; and 2 females, ages 8 and 10 years). Of these, 9 (60 percent) had preexisting tics before stimulant medication was begun. Of the 15, 8 had a family history of tics or Tourette's disorder. In most cases the Tourette's disorder did not remit following discontinuation of stimulants, and medication was required to control the Tourette's disorder. These authors strongly recommended that stimulants are contraindicated in treating ADDH in children with tics or Tourette's disorder. They suggest that stimulants should be used with great caution when there is a family history of tics or Tourette's disorder, and should be discontinued immediately if tics develop while a child is on stimulants regardless of family history.

Others, however, disagree and conclude that stimulants probably do not significantly accelerate the development of Tourette's disorder (Shapiro & Shapiro, 1981) or suggest that patients who develop tics on stimulants probably have a genetic predisposition and would have developed tics without having received stimulant medication (Comings & Comings, 1984).

Growth and Stimulant Medication

There has been concern since the early 1970s that stimulants adversely affect both linear growth and weight in children. Quinn and

Rapoport (1975) reported that 23 boys who had been on methyl-phenidate (mean daily dose, 20.65 ± 8.56) lost about 8.8 percentile points in weight (p < .005) and gained about 3.2 percentile points (N.S.) in height. The 5 boys receiving over 20 mg methylphenidate or less daily showed a 15.4 percentile weight loss (p < .005) and a 3.0 percentile height decrease (N.S.), whereas the 18 boys receiving 20 mg or less daily of methylphenidate showed only 6.88 percentile points loss in weight (p < .005) and a 5.12 gain in height percentile (p < .05).

McNutt et al. (1976) conducted a prospective study of 26 hyperactive children who received methylphenidate 0.3-1.86 mg/kg/day (mean 0.59 mg/kg/day) for two years. Their weights and heights did not differ significantly from controls.

Satterfield et al. (1979) studied growth in a prospective study in hyperactive boys between ages 6 and 12 treated with methylphenidate. For one year 72 were followed; 48 were followed for two years. There was an adverse effect on both weight and height during the first year. During the second year, mean weight gain was 0.31 kg less and mean height gain was 0.42 cm more than expected. These were not signifi-cantly different from expected values. Height gain in the second year was sufficient to make up for the loss during the first year. The authors concluded that reduction of height and weight growth rates by methylphenidate was temporary and of such minor magnitude (less than 1 percent deficit in expected adult height) that it had little clinical significance.

The Pediatric Subcommittee of the Food and Drug Administration Psychopharmacologic Drugs Advisory Committee (Roche et al., 1979) reviewed the available data on growth suppression by stimulant medications in prepubertal hyperkinetic children. They concluded that in the "high dose" range (e.g., methylphenidate > 20 mg/day) stimulants moderately suppress growth in weight. Although there may be minor suppression of linear growth, it is no longer evident in adulthood.

At variance with the former conclusion is the report of Mattes and Gittelman (1983). They studied growth in 86 hyperactive children who were maintained on an average dose of 40 mg of methylphenidate daily for up to four years. Height percentiles progressively decreased from 1.4 percentile points below expectation after the first year (not significant) to an 18.1 percentile decrease (p < .001) after four years. There was also a significant decrease in weight percentile over the four-year period (p < .001). A subgroup of 34 children who received thioridazine concurrently with methylphenidate did not differ significantly in their growth rates from those children who received methylphenidate only.

In view of the discrepant results of the above studies it is evident that some children may be at greater risk for growth suppression than others. Careful longitudinal monitoring of height and weight percentiles is indicated.

4

TRICYCLIC ANTIDEPRESSANTS

INDICATIONS

Currently, imipramine is the most widely prescribed drug for the treatment of functional enuresis in childhood; it can be a useful intervention in its short-term management or situational treatment (e.g., overnight outings). However, long-term utilization of imipramine on a routine basis for this indication is not advised, because more effective and less invasive interventions are available (e.g., bell-and-pad conditioning; McConaghy, 1969; Rapoport, Mikkelsen et al., 1980). When enuresis appears as a regressive symptom, its cause should be identified, rather than simply masked with imipramine. Moreover, a substantial number of boys who demonstrate an initial antienuretic effect from imipramine sometimes develop tolerance after prolonged administration (Rapoport, Mikkelsen et al., 1980). In the evaluation of enuresis, an etiology should be sought prior to the initiation of treatment. In most individuals, enuresis will spontaneously resolve without any intervention (Forsythe & Redmond, 1974). The routine use of imipramine for enuresis cannot be endorsed because of the efficacy of psychosocial interventions and, furthermore, because of its toxicity.

Imipramine may also play a role in the management of hyperkinesis. The failure of individual hyperactive patients to respond to stimulant medications has prompted interest in imipramine as an alternative agent, and there appears to be a subgroup of hyperactive children who are imipramine responders. However, tolerance to imipramine's salutary effects has been reported in some hyperactive and aggressive children (Quinn & Rapoport, 1975).

In conjunction with psychosocial interventions involving parents, child, and school authorities, imipramine may play an important role in the treatment of school phobia (Gittelman-Klein & Klein, 1973a).

The identification of prepubertal children who fulfill unmodified adult criteria for major depressive disorder (MDD) led to antidepressant trials in children with this condition. The results of several studies support the responsiveness of prepubertal depression to imipramine and suggest a continuity between these disorders in children and adults. Adolescent depressives are less responsive to imipramine; this may be due to an antagonistic effect of estrogen (Puig-Antich, 1984).

Imipramine may be a useful drug for some electrophysiologic disorders associated with stages 3 and 4 of sleep, particularly pavor nocturnus and somnambulism (Pesikoff & Davis, 1971).

A readjustment of neural transmission along noradrenergic and serotonergic pathways, due to subsensitization of beta-noradrenergic and serotonin receptors, has been postulated to mediate the therapeutic response to chronic antidepressant administration (Charney et al., 1981). Indirectly, norepinephrine and serotonin are implicated in disorders that benefit from tricyclic antidepressants. Although the receptor desensitization model may account for the efficacy of these drugs in relieving depression, it might not account for the efficacy of tricyclics in hyperkinesis; in the latter condition, the clinical response to the tricyclic occurs as soon as a therapeutically effective dose is attained, and the effect wears off within a few days after the tricyclic is discontinued (Huessy & Wright, 1970). The ensuing review will selectively examine seminal studies relating to tricyclic antidepressant efficacy in enuresis, hyperactivity and aggressiveness, school phobia, major depressive disorder, pavor nocturnus, and somnambulism (for summary see Table 4).

CONTRAINDICATIONS

Imipramine is contraindicated in children with cardiac conduction abnormalities or children receiving medications that affect cardiac conduction or repolarization. Tricyclic antidepressants should be used with caution in seizure-prone individuals or children receiving antiseizure medications. Finally, in the absence of major depression, they are not recommended for psychotic children as they can worsen psychotic disorganization.

DOSAGE

Imipramine is prescribed in doses of 25 to 50 mg h.s. in the treatment of nocturnal enuresis in children aged 6 years and older. A dosage of 2.5 mg/kg/day should not be exceeded. The status of imipramine in the treatment of depression and behavior disorders in children is viewed as investigational. The FDA has presented guidelines for investigational protocols of imipramine hydrochloride in children. Only those protocols that do not exceed the following maximum daily dosages, based on weight, will be approved: 90 mg/40-lb child, 110 mg/50-lb child, 135 mg/60-lb child, 160 mg/70-lb child, and 180 mg/80-lb child (about 2.2 mg/lb. These guidelines also include regular EKG monitoring as maximum dosages are approached (Hayes et al., 1975).

SHORT- AND LONG-TERM EFFICACY

Effect on Behavioral Symptoms

Enuresis. The antienuretic efficacy of imipramine was studied in 47 high-frequency nocturnally enuretic children (ages 5 to 16 years) (Poussaint & Ditman, 1965). This outpatient study lasted eight weeks and employed a double-blind placebo-controlled design. In all children, the frequency of enuresis was greater than once per week. No obvious organic etiology could account for the persistent enuresis. During the eight-week trial, dosages of imipramine were fixed: 25 mg for children under 12 years and 50 mg for children 12 years and older. Medication was given one-half to one hour before bedtime and "wet" and "dry" nights were recorded. There were four groups as follows: (1) imipramine (4 weeks), placebo (4 weeks), n = 13; (2) placebo (4 weeks), imipramine (4 weeks), n = 13; (3) imipramine (8 weeks), n = 10; and (4) placebo (8 weeks), n = 11. In the 26 crossover patients, imipramine was significantly superior to placebo in decreasing the frequency of enuretic nights (p < .0005). Irrespective of treatment group, all children showed a decrease in the frequency of their bed-wetting compared with pretreatment values. Although the difference did not achieve statistical significance, noncrossover patients receiving imipramine (Group 3) showed an aver-

TABLE 4 Representative Studies of Tricyclic Antidepressants in Childhood Disorders

Tricyclic Antidepressant	Indication	Dosage	Comments	Authors
Imipramine	Enuresis	Max. dose 50 mg (ages 5 to 7 years) Max. dose 75 mg (ages ⩾ 10 years)	Positive antienuretic effect.	Poussaint & Ditman (1965)
Imipramine	Enuresis	75 mg at bedtime	Positive short-term antienuretic effect; subgroups of transient responders and nonresponders were identified.	Rapoport et al. (1980)
Desipramine	Enuresis	75 mg at bedtime	Positive short-term antienuretic effect.	Rapoport et al. (1980)
Imipramine	Hyperactivity and learning disability	10 to 40 mg/day	Improved attention span, ability to concentrate, and academic performance—a noncontrolled open-label study.	Rapoport (1965)
Imipramine	Hyperkinetic syndrome and learning difficulty	25 to 125 mg/day (mean 50)	High response rate and convenient dosage schedule. Parents and school reported improvement.	Huessy & Wright (1970)
Imipramine	Hyperactivity and aggressiveness	75 to 150 mg/day	Decreased hyperactivity and aggressiveness. Improved attention span (a short-term 7 to 10 day trial).	Winsberg et al. (1972)

Imipramine	Hyperactivity	Mean dosage 80 mg/day	Positive therapeutic effects; methylphenidate superior to imipramine.	Rapoport et al. (1974)
Imipramine	Hyperactivity	Mean dosage 65.4 mg/day	A one-year follow-up study. High rate of discontinuation; development of tolerance observed. In responders, equieffective to methylphenidate.	Quinn & Rapoport (1975)
Imipramine	Hyperactivity	100 to 200 mg/day (mean 173.7)	Positive therapeutic effects.	Waizer et al. (1974)
Imipramine	Hyperactivity	1.0 mg/kg/day versus 2.0 mg/kg/day	Positive therapeutic effects. Low dosage as effective as high dosage.	Werry et al. (1980)
Imipramine	School Phobia	100 to 200 mg/day (mean 152)	Positive therapeutic effects.	Gittelman-Klein & Klein (1973)
Imipramine	Depression	Max. dosage between 4 and 5 mg/kg/day	Positive therapeutic effects.	Puig-Antich et al. (1978)
Imipramine	Depression	75 mg at bedtime	Positive therapeutic effects observed in 80% to 90% of children with plasma levels above 125 ng/mL. Many children on this fixed dose had sub-therapeutic plasma levels.	Weller et al. (1982)
Imipramine	Depression	75 mg at bedtime for 3 weeks; thereafter, dosage was individually regulated (max. 5 mg/kg/day).	Therapeutic range of plasma levels between 125-225 ng/mL	Preskorn et al. (1982); Weller et al. (1983)

(continued)

TABLE 4 Continued

Tricyclic Antidepressant	Indication	Dosage	Comments	Authors
Imipramine	Depression	Max. dosage 5 mg/kg/day	Positive therapeutic effects.	Petti & Law (1982)
Imipramine	Depression	Max. dosage 5 mg/kg/day	85% of children with plasma levels above 155 ng/ml showed a positive therapeutic response. Oral dosage could not be used to predict clinical response. Children with severe or psychotic symptoms were less sensitive to imipramine; they required higher plasma levels.	Puig-Antich et al. (1979; in press)
Nortriptyline	Depression	20 to 50 mg/day	Positive therapeutic effects.	Geller et al. (1983)
Amitriptyline	Depression	Fixed dose 1.5 mg/kg/day; dosage range 45 to 110 mg/day	Positive therapeutic effects.	Kashani et al. (1984)
Imipramine	Sleep disorders— Pavor Nocturnus and Somnambulism	10 to 50 mg at bedtime	Positive therapeutic effects.	Pesikoff & Davis (1971)

age net difference of about two more dry nights per week at the end of the eighth week than the noncrossover patients receiving placebo (Group 4). At the end of the study, 6 children receiving imipramine were completely dry as contrasted with only 1 child receiving placebo. After the conclusion of the double-blind trial, 46 of the children were followed on imipramine on an open basis; dosage was regulated on an individual basis. Maximum allowable dosage was 75 mg for children 10 years and older; children between the ages of 5 and 7 years were not increased beyond 50 mg. Many children for whom the dosage was increased showed a dramatic positive antienuretic response. The antienuretic response of 39 out of 46 children (85 percent) was at least marked; in 11 patients, a complete remission was maintained after gradual withdrawal from a two-month course on optimal dosages of medication. Only 7 patients remained nonresponders to the antienuretic action of imipramine during the open phase of the study. The authors were not impressed with the development of tolerance to the antienuretic action of imipramine.

The antienuretic efficacy of imipramine (75 mg at bedtime) was compared with desipramine (75 mg at bedtime) and methscopolamine (6 mg at bedtime) in two separate double-blind crossover studies involving a total of 40 nocturnally enuretic boys (ages 7 to 12 years; mean 10.8 ± 1.5 [SD] years) (Rapoport, Mikkelsen et al., 1980). These crossover comparisons were preceded by a ten-day phase of placebo administration during which the parents and children were blind to the nature of the medication. In all subjects, the frequency of enuresis was at least five nights per week for the year preceding study enrollment. The outpatient trials at home lasted a total of ten days and, with the inclusion of the inpatient studies, drugs were prescribed for periods of fifteen days. At the end of the ten-day outpatient trials, the children were admitted for sleep recordings. After each active medication period, blood samples were obtained for determination of plasma tricyclic levels. Methscopolamine is a peripherally acting anticholinergic agent that does not cross the blood-brain barrier; desipramine has lesser anticholinergic and greater adrenergic activity than imipramine. With the inclusion of these drugs, the relative contribution of peripheral cholinergic blockade and central adrenergic activation to imipramine's antienuretic action could be determined. Imipramine and desipramine were significantly superior to placebo in increasing the frequency of dry nights in ten nights of treatment. Neither antidepressant differed significantly from the other. Children treated with either methscopolamine or placebo did not differ in terms of frequency of nocturnal enuresis. Thus antienuretic efficacy did not appear to be due to peripheral cholinergic blockade. Most boys were only "partial responders" to either antidepressant— complete cessation of enuresis occurred only rarely. The tricyclics decreased the frequency of enuretic episodes during the night but did not alter the time of their occurrence. These investigators had reported that no significant relationship existed between enuretic episodes and sleep stages (Mikkelsen et al., 1980). Thus the antienuretic effects of the tricyclics are not likely to be due to their alteration of sleep stages (Rapoport, Mikkelsen et al., 1980). Drug conditions were not associated with any changes in the behavioral ratings. In terms of plasma tricyclic levels, wide interindividual variability was observed (Rapoport, Mikkelsen et al., 1980). Significant positive relationships between plasma levels of desipramine, plasma levels of desipramine plus imipramine, and continence were observed. Antienuretic responses were observed with plasma levels of desipramine or total (desipramine plus imipramine) tricyclic antidepressant at or above 150 ng/ml.

At the conclusion of the short-term study, treatment was individualized and most of the boys received imipramine on an open basis. Follow-up of 36 imipramine-treated children at least one month after completion of the short-term study revealed the existence of three groups: good responders (n = 17), nonresponders (n = 6) and transient responders (n = 13). Transient responders showed an initial good response during the short-term study but became tolerant to the antienuretic effects with continued treatment. Plasma levels obtained on some of the follow-up children showed that transient responsiveness or nonresponsiveness occurred despite "adequate" plasma levels. These data suggest that subgroups of enuretic children who are not responsive to imipramine exist and that tolerance can develop to the antienuretic effect (Rapoport, Mikkelsen et al., 1980).

Hyperactivity and other behavioral symptoms. In 1965, Rapoport summarized his clinical experiences with relatively low-dose imipramine therapy administered to a heterogeneous group of 41 private patients (ages 5 to 21 years). The majority of these patients were in early adolescence and demonstrated subtle electroencephalographic abnormalities. They presented with a varied constellation of symptoms: restlessness, distractibility, impulsivity, temper tantrums, frank delinquency, daydreaming, and poor learning abilities. As they were not amenable to dynamically-oriented therapies, the value of medication selected on an empirical basis was investigated. Imipramine was initiated at a dosage of 10 mg at bedtime and maximal dosages were 40 mg/day; most patients were maintained on 20 mg/day. The trials to determine effectiveness lasted from four to six weeks. In responders, the duration of active treatment ranged from 6 months to 2 years (mean 12 months). On a qualitative basis, 33 patients (80.5 percent) showed a good response to treatment. This early report suffered from many methodological inadequacies; most notable were the absence of specified diagnostic criteria, non-blind design and the absence of objective outcome measures.

The beneficial effects of imipramine, administered on an open basis, prompted a more systematic study of its efficacy in the "hyperkinetic syndrome" (Huessy & Wright, 1970). Imipramine was administered on an individually regulated basis to 52 children (sex ratio 3 boys: 1 girl; ages 3 to 14 years) referred by physicians because of hyperkinesis and behavior that was interfering with school functioning or family life. All of these children were of normal intelligence and shared at least three of twelve defined diagnostic criteria. Imipramine was initiated according to dosage guidelines based on age and weight; medication was increased at three day intervals. Trials to determine the presence of any positive drug effects lasted two weeks. Children were determined to show a positive response to medication only if parents and school reported "marked and definite improvement in behavior and performance." A total of 35 children (67 percent) were responders and their dosage ranged from 25 to 125 mg/day (mean 50). In most cases, imipramine was administered as a convenient single dose about one-half to one hour before bedtime. Therapeutic effects, if present, were observed the following day. After four months of continuous administration to responders, medication was stopped to determine the need for continued treatment. When medication was stopped after four months, the majority of children showed a reemergence of premedication behaviors. Only 2 children (4 percent) continued to do well without medication. In the others, improvement was again observed with reinitiation of imipramine and therapeutic efficacy persisted for 12 to 18 months at the time of this report. Some of the more verbal children reported subjective improvement from taking the medication. A child requesting medication after its discontinuation at four months said, "it unscrambles my brain." Due to the relatively high percentage of responders (67 percent) and the convenience of one daily evening dosage, these authors have selected imipramine as their drug of first choice in the treatment of the hyperkinetic syndrome (Huessy & Wright, 1970). Tolerance to imipramine's therapeutic effects was not observed in this study.

Over a six-month period, open administration of imipramine to a group of behavior disordered children resulted in attenuation of hyperactivity and aggressiveness without liver or hematologic toxicity (Winsberg et al., 1972). These observations prompted a short term controlled outpatient study comparing the effectiveness of imipramine with dextroamphetamine and placebo (Winsberg et al., 1972). The study sample, which consisted of 32 children (26 boys and 6 girls), was heterogeneous with respect to age (63 months to 163 months) and IQ (40 to 113). Most children were diagnosed as hyperkinetic reaction or minimal cerebral dysfunction; however, the diagnostic criteria were not specified. The remaining diagnoses included childhood schizophrenia and diagnosis deferred or uncertain. All of the children shared the same serious referral complaints, for instance, "either aggressive behavior or hyperactivity of sufficient proportion to warrant chemotherapy for the control of these behaviors." Children were assigned to one of two counterbalanced sequences of medication conditions: imipramine-placebo-dextroamphetamine or dextroamphetamine-placebo-imipramine. Each condition lasted from seven to ten days. Parents administered the medication in a double-blind fashion: 5 or 10 mg of dextroamphetamine three times a day, 25 or 50 mg of imipramine three times a day, and one placebo tablet three times a day. In some instances, medication was adjusted either because of side effects or absence of response. Using a 39-item behavior rating scale (Conners, 1969), parents rated the frequency of a variety of behaviors prior to the start of the protocol and at the end of each medication condition. Imipramine and dextroamphetamine were shown to reduce mean summed factor scores for aggressivity and hyperactivity significantly; only imipramine was able to reduce inattention. In terms of individual responsivity, a greater number of children were sensitive to the positive effects of imipramine than dextroamphetamine. In view of the fact that mutually exclusive subgroups of children who responded either to imipramine alone (n = 12) or dextroamphetamine alone (n = 4) were identified, imipramine may be useful as an alternative agent in stimulant nonresponders. Clinically, the authors noted that the phenomenon of tolerance to drug effects was observed.

In an outpatient study involving 76 boys (ages 6 to 12 years) referred for persistent distractibility or motor restlessness and impulsivity, imipramine was compared with methylphenidate and placebo in a double-blind noncrossover design of six weeks duration (Rapoport et al., 1974). All children were of normal intelligence (IQ $\geq$ 80), from middle-class families, and free of any known neurological disorder. Children were assigned to one of three treatment groups: methylphenidate (n = 29), imipramine (n = 29), and placebo (n = 18). Medication or placebo was individually regulated according to the emergence of side effects or lack of response. The maximum imipramine and methylphenidate dosage permitted any child was 150 mg/day and 30 mg/day, respectively. Mean imipramine and methylphenidate dosages were 80 mg/day and 20 mg/day, respectively. Both drugs were viewed as effective, but methylphenidate was judged to be superior and was associated with less prominent side effects. Global ratings of change at six weeks by the physician showed that imipramine was superior to placebo (p < .001), although it was significantly less effective than methylphenidate (p < .02). The psychologist was less impressed with the magnitude of any positive drug effects; globally, he rated the children receiving methylphenidate as improved compared with placebo (p < .05) but imipramine was indistinguishable statistically from placebo. With both drugs, parents and teachers recorded a diminution of "impulsive-hyperactive" and "hyperactivity" factor scores on the Conners Parent and Teacher Rating Scales, respectively. Although the percentage of improvement was not as pronounced as with methylphenidate, the teacher's global ratings of change in classroom behavior and academic achievement showed greater improvement with imipramine than with placebo. According to the psychologist's ratings, the children receiving imipramine showed a diminution of attentional difficulties as compared with placebo. Suboptimal imipramine dosage, as reflected in subtherapeutic plasma levels, could have accounted for the failure to observe greater imipramine efficacy.

Follow-up data after one year were obtained on 75 of the original 76 hyperactive boys who participated in the six-week comparison trial of imipramine with methylphenidate and placebo (Quinn & Rapoport, 1975). After the initial six-week trial, the boys in the placebo group were randomly assigned to a nonblind six-week trial of either imipramine or methylphenidate. All responders were encouraged to remain on active medication. For purposes of comparison, a group of 12 boys, who initially responded to medication but discontinued treatment within four months because of parental concerns over side effects or drug use, was identified. After one year, the mean imipramine dosage was 65.4 mg/day $\pm$ 19.2 (SD) and only 18 of 37 boys continued to receive imipramine following their initial trial. Thus about 51 percent of the imipramine group discontinued their medication as contrasted with a 24 percent rate of methylphenidate discontinuation. The reasons for imipramine discontinuation included unchanged behavior, hypertension, irritability and temper tantrums, and parental disapproval. Despite drug treatment, few of the follow-up children were viewed as symptom-free at one year. However, at one year, a comparison of imipramine-treated boys (n = 13), methylphenidate-treated boys (n = 23), and boys discontinued from medication (n = 12) showed that both drugs were equally effective in significantly reducing the mean summed conduct and hyperactivity factor scores on the Teacher Rating Scale. The three groups could not be distinguished using the parental ratings. Although significantly fewer children tolerated imipramine than methylphenidate (p < .01), in children maintained on these drugs for one year, they were equally effective and superior to no treatment in improving classroom behavior. These results were not seen by parents in the less structured home environment. The imposition of structure may elicit or exacerbate the target behaviors in hyperactive children.

The reports of salutary effects of imipramine prompted an eight-week outpatient study of imipramine's effectiveness in 19 hyperkinetic boys (ages 6 to 12 years; Waizer et al., 1974). All children were diagnosed as hyperkinetic reaction of childhood according to DSM II (American Psychiatric Association, 1968). Upon enrollment, children were maintained drug free for at least one week prior to receiving an eight-week trial of imipramine followed by a four-week trial of placebo. At regular intervals, as well as after the one-week baseline period, assessments were performed by the treating psychiatrist, teachers, and parents. Parents and teachers served as blind observers. Imipramine was initiated at a dosage of 50 mg/day and, thereafter, it was individually regulated. The final dosages ranged from 100 to 200 mg/day (mean 173.7) and in most cases were administered at bedtime. In terms of the psychiatrist's global rating, 14 children were viewed as much improved and two showed minimal improvement by the eighth week of imipramine treatment. This was also reflected in a reduction of the mean score on the 19-item scale filled out by the psychiatrist. The Hyperactivity List completed by parents reflected clinical improvement in hyperactivity; however, significant improvement was not shown with the Conners Parent Symptom Questionnaire. Teachers recognized improvement by the second week of imipramine treatment, as reflected in their global impressions and significant reductions in mean scores of four factors (hyperactivity, defiance, inattentiveness, and sociability) on the Conners Teacher Rating Scale. Although behaviors worsened during the placebo period, there was the suggestion of some sustained improvement.

The efficacy of two dosage levels of imipramine (1.0 and 2.0 mg/kg/day) was compared with a fixed dosage of methylphenidate (0.40 mg/kg/day) and placebo in a double-blind crossover design involving 30 hyperactive children (26 boys and 4 girls; ages 5 years, 6 months to 12 years, 7 months; Werry et al., 1980). The fixed methylphenidate dosage selected in this study was shown previously to improve behaviors and learning. The children were randomly assigned to one of two counterbalanced orders of drug conditions: imipramine-placebo-methylphenidate or methylphenidate-placebo-imipramine. At a dosage of 1.0 mg/kg/day, 14 of the children received imipramine in their first drug condition, whereas 16 children received an imipramine dosage of 2.0 mg/kg/day in their last drug condition. Each drug condition lasted for a period of at least three and up to four weeks. A variety of measures was obtained prior to treatment and after each of the drug conditions.

Order of drug administration was not found to be significant. On the physician's global ratings of improvement, imipramine was unexpectedly found to be superior to methylphenidate. The clinical superiority of imipramine was also reflected in the Conners Parent Symptom Questionnaire; as opposed to methylphenidate or placebo, imipramine improved mean summed factor scores for conduct and hyperactivity. However, no significant effect of either drug was shown on the Conners Teacher Rating Scale. Seat movement was recorded as a measure of motor activity and was reduced significantly by both active medications. No increased therapeutic benefit of imipramine was observed with the higher dosage. In this study, the therapeutic efficacy of imipramine was superior to methylphenidate and placebo. However, the physician's reliance upon parental reports may have biased global assessments in favor of imipramine. With a short-acting drug like methylphenidate, positive effects may wane by the time a child arrives home from school. In this respect, the relative insensitivity of the Teacher Rating Scale to drug effects in this study was unfortunate.

In summary, the results of several independent studies justify a trial of imipramine in stimulant-nonresponsive hyperactive children.

School phobia. In a double-blind placebo-controlled study of six weeks duration, the effectiveness of imipramine was examined in the treatment of 35 school phobic children (16 boys and 19 girls, ages 6 to 14 years; Gittelman-Klein & Klein, 1973a). The efficacy of imipramine in the treatment of school phobia was examined because of the beneficial effects of this drug in adult patients with phobic disorders and panic attacks. Marked separation anxiety and difficulty with school adjustment, including phobic reactions, were elicited in the childhood histories of many of these adult patients. The children were randomly assigned to one of two treatment conditions: drug (n = 16) or matching placebo (n = 19). Imipramine was given in two divided doses and followed a fixed dosage regimen for the first two weeks; dosage was 75 mg/day during the second week. Thereafter, it was individually regulated on a weekly basis and ranged from 100 to 200 mg/day (mean = 152) at the end of six weeks. Assessments were performed on baseline and after three and six weeks of treatment. Despite a high placebo response rate, imipramine was significantly superior to placebo in terms of improved school attendance at the end of six weeks. However, using school attendance as the outcome measure, there was a lag before therapeutic efficacy was observed because imipramine and placebo did not differ after three weeks. In terms of global improvement, all of the imipramine-treated children reported that they were much improved after six weeks; mothers and psychiatrists reported that they showed significantly greater improvement than the placebo-treated children.

Depression. The results of several well-controlled studies support the clinical efficacy of imipramine in the treatment of prepubertal depression. Efficacy appears to be related to plasma levels of imipramine and/or its demethylated metabolite, desipramine; plasma levels cannot be predicted from the oral dosage. In depressed children fulfilling DSM III (American Psychiatric Association, 1980) criteria for MDD, approximately 90 percent respond positively with plasma tricyclic levels above 155 ng/ml (Puig-Antich et al., 1979; Puig-Antich et al., in press). The response rate of adolescent depressives to imipramine is lower—about 40 percent (Puig-Antich, 1984). This lowered sensitivity among adolescents could be due to an antagonistic effect of estrogen. The safety and efficacy of monoamine oxidase inhibitors have not been carefully studied in children. Studies exploring tricyclic antidepressant efficacy in prepubertal depression will be reviewed.

The clinical responses of eight prepubertal children (ages 6 to 12 years) who fulfilled unmodified adult Research Diagnostic Criteria (RCD) (Spitzer et al., 1978) for MDD to three to four weeks of treatment with imipramine were examined in an open-label pilot study

(Puig-Antich et al., 1978). Imipramine was initiated at a dose of 1.5 mg/kg/day administered in three divided doses. Increments of 1.5 mg/kg/day occurred about weekly and, barring severe side effects, maximum dosage was to be between 4 and 5 mg/kg/day in all children. After four continuous weeks on maximum dosage, 6 of 8 children were responders. The availability of blood levels in some patients explained the positive response of a 7-year old girl to a relatively low dosage and the failure of one of the two nonresponders receiving a relatively high dosage. In the responder receiving a low dosage (2 mg/kg/day), her dramatic response was attributed to a placebo effect until a plasma total tricyclic level of 194 ng/ml was determined. In adults, this level is within the therapeutic range. The nonresponder in whom plasma tricyclic levels were obtained was a 10-year old girl who fulfilled criteria for a psychotic subtype and who failed to respond to a dosage of 4 mg/kg/day. Even at this relatively high dosage, her plasma level was 100 ng/ml. In adults, this level is below or at the lower end of the therapeutic range. After the trial, her dosage was increased to 5 mg/kg/day and her plasma total tricyclic level was raised to 304 ng/ml. At this dose, her depression remitted in two weeks. Although somnolence and dry mouth necessitated dosage reduction, her remission was maintained at a dose of 4.5 mg/kg/day.

In order to examine a possible reason for varying response rates to imipramine, steady-state plasma tricyclic levels on a fixed bedtime dose of imipramine were examined in 11 hospitalized boys (ages 7 to 12 years) fulfilling DSM III (1980) criteria for MDD (Weller et al., 1982). Imipramine was initiated and maintained at a fixed dose of 75 mg at bedtime in order to obtain information regarding interindividual variability of plasma tricyclic levels. In these 11 boys, there was a sixfold variation in combined imipramine and desipramine steady-state plasma levels ranging from 56 to 324 ng/ml, despite the same 75-mg oral dose. Levels of the demethylated active metabolite exceeded those of the parent compound with ratios ranging from 1.2 to 3.5. Dosage could not be titrated according to age, height, weight, or body surface area to ensure therapeutic plasma concentrations. Five children who failed to respond to the fixed imipramine dosage after three weeks had total plasma levels below 125 ng/ml. Upon dosage increase, these "nonresponders" responded when their plasma concentrations rose above 125 ng/ml. The only patient experiencing distressing side effects had a total plasma concentration of 324 ng/ml on the fixed 75-mg dosage. Side effects disappeared and the depression improved when the dosage was reduced to 50 mg/day. The results emphasize the importance of measuring plasma levels in the evaluation of patients who either fail to respond or who manifest severe and dose-limiting side effects while receiving "therapeutic" dosages of imipramine.

The relationship between therapeutic response and plasma tricyclic concentrations was assessed in 20 hospitalized children (16 boys and 4 girls; ages 7 to 12 years) fulfilling DSM III (1980) criteria for MDD (Preskorn et al., 1982; Weller et al., 1983). The children were treated with a fixed 75-mg h.s. dose of imipramine for three weeks in an open-label study. Patients who failed to respond to the fixed 75-mg h.s. imipramine dose after three weeks were eligible for three additional weeks of treatment on an individually titrated dose. In the second three-week phase, the dosage was reduced to 50 mg/day in nonresponders with side effects and increased to a maximum of 5 mg/kg/day in nonresponders without side effects. A subset of 4 of 5 children with steady-state plasma total tricyclic concentrations in the range of 125 to 225 ng/ml experienced a remission after three weeks of continuous treatment on the fixed 75-mg h.s. dose of imipramine. Another child with levels in this range after the same amount of time on the fixed 75-mg h.s. dose regimen showed marked improvement but did not meet the objective criteria for remission. On the fixed imipramine dose of 75 mg at bedtime, 11 children had plasma total tricyclic concentrations below 125 ng/ml. Thus 55 percent of the sample had plasma tricyclic levels below the minimum therapeutic level. If only those children with total plasma tricyclic levels in the range of 125-225 ng/ml are considered, then an 80 percent remission rate was observed after three weeks. The investigators found curvilinear relationships between the antidepressant response and the plasma concentrations of total tricyclic and desipramine alone. No similar relationship between antidepressant response and plasma imipramine concentration was detected. Thus there may be a maximum plasma total tricyclic level (> 225 ng/ml) above which therapeutic effects are not observed (therapeutic window), and therapeutic effects may be primarily due to desipramine.

Sixteen children entered the second three-week drug treatment phase of the study. At the end of this phase, 11 of 12 children (92 percent) with plasma total tricyclic levels in the range of 125 to 225 ng/ml experienced remission. One child who received six weeks of continuous treatment remitted with plasma levels below the therapeutic range. Thus in addition to plasma levels, duration of treatment is another factor contributing to therapeutic response.

In a pilot study involving 6 hospitalized prepubertal depressed children (5 boys and 1 girl; ages 6 to 12 years), imipramine was compared with placebo using double-blind procedures, random assignment of patients to drug and placebo conditions, and standardized rating instruments (Petti & Law, 1982). All 6 children fulfilled criteria for the retrospective assignment of MDD according to DSM III (1980). The two groups of 3 children entered a six-week period of treatment with either imipramine or placebo. At the end of the first week, dosage was increased to maximum—approximately 5 mg/kg/day. The maximum dosage was maintained for three weeks. Medication was slowly tapered during the fifth week and stopped during the last week of the study. All 3 imipramine-treated children showed evidence of at least mild improvement, whereas 2 of the 3 placebo-treated children worsened. Interestingly, the imipramine-treated child who displayed "only subjective mild clinical improvement" had the highest plasma tricyclic levels (total = 385.6 ng/ml). This isolated observation is consistent with the existence of a therapeutic window. Blood for these levels was drawn during the three-week maintenance phase. Nevertheless, the less responsive imipramine-treated child did show steady improvement and eventual remission. Subsequent to the completion of the study, all placebo-treated children received imipramine and responded with relief of their depression.

In order to identify predictors of clinical response and clarify the relationship between maintenance plasma tricyclic levels and clinical response, 30 prepubertal patients (18 boys and 12 girls, mean age 9.56 ± 1.46 years) fulfilling unmodified RDC for adult MDD were treated for five weeks with maintenance doses of imipramine (Puig-Antich et al., 1979; in press). Imipramine was initiated at a dosage of 1.5 mg/kg/day, in three divided doses, with increments occurring at three-day intervals to a maximum of 5 mg/kg/day. The protocol of dosage administration was fixed and independent of the severity of depressive symptomatology. Increments were not made if severe side effects or cardiac abnormalities emerged. Weekly EKGs were obtained to monitor cardiac status. Children were maintained at maximum doses for five weeks. At the end of the five weeks, treatment response was assessed with administration of the Schedule for Affective Disorders and Schizophrenia for School Age Children (Kiddie-SADS), focusing on the period covering the entire fifth week, by a rater who was blind to plasma levels. Blood samples to determine maintenance plasma levels were obtained at the end of weeks 2, 3, 4, and 5. The results paralleled observations in adults: Mean maintenance total plasma levels were higher in responders than nonresponders (p < .007). Of children with plasma levels over 155 ng/ml, 85 percent responded positively to imipramine, as contrasted with only 30 percent of children responding with levels below this amount (p < .009). No relationship existed between response and oral imipramine dosage on a mg/kg basis. Thus, oral dosage was a poor predictor of clinical response. Children with more severe or psychotic symptoms required higher plasma levels to achieve a positive clinical response. A positive response was likely to occur if levels of either imipramine or desipramine were above their median values (60 and 110.5 ng/ml, respectively). In more than half of the children, imipramine could not be raised to the maximum allowable dosage of 5 mg/kg/day. The limiting side effects included lengthening of PR interval (n = 9); heart rate above 130/min (n = 1); orthostatic hypotension (n = 2); marked irritability (n = 2); chest pain (n = 1); and forgetfulness and perplexity (n = 2). In conclusion, imipramine was an effective drug when plasma total levels exceeded 155 ng/ml at the steady state. Oral dosage could not be used to predict clinical response.

The rate of hepatic demethylation of imipramine is faster in children than adults. Geller and her associates (1983) reasoned that the therapeutic efficacy of imipramine could be largely attributable to its active metabolite, desipramine. Desipramine is a secondary, predominantly noradrenergic, tricyclic antidepressant. Therefore, these investigators examined the efficacy of a predominantly noradrenergic antidepressant (Geller et al., 1983). They selected nortriptyline because of the safety of this compound in a high-risk geriatric population and the fact that predictive kinetics, pharmacokinetics, therapeutic range, and stability of plasma levels are well established in adults. Nortriptyline is the demethylated metabolite of amitriptyline. On an open basis, nortriptyline was administered to 12 prepubertal children (8 boys and 4 girls, ages 5 to 11 years) with MDD for a total treatment period of 16 weeks. Most of the children responded in 2 to 8 weeks on continuous dosages of 20 to 50 mg/day. Four subjects relapsed during weeks 13 and 14 in the maintenance phase of the study. In these 4 children, plasma nortriptyline levels fell below the therapeutic range. Optimal dosage could be predicted from plasma nortriptyline levels occurring 48 hours after the administration of a single 25-mg oral dose. The half-life of the drug was over 12 hours, suggesting that twice daily dosage be employed to ensure stable plasma levels. Serious side effects were not observed and in only 2 children were transient EKG abnormalities seen; EKG abnormalities occurred when plasma nortriptyline levels exceeded the adult therapeutic range.

In the long-term administration of amitriptyline, plasma levels of the parent tertiary—predominantly serotonergic—compound often exceed those of the active demethylated metabolite. Thus amitriptyline may possess greater efficacy than imipramine in depressions with a relatively greater deficiency of central serotonergic transmission. The efficacy of amitriptyline was examined in a fixed dose double-blind crossover pilot study involving 9 prepubertal depressed inpatients (8 boys and 1 girl, ages 9 to 12 years; Kashani et al., 1984). The children were selected according to the DSM III (1980) criteria for MDD. Dosage was initiated at 1 mg/kg/day, in three divided doses, and raised to the maintenance and fixed level of 1.5 mg/kg/day after 3 days. After four weeks of treatment with either amitriptyline or placebo, the drug condition was switched to four weeks of alternate treatment. The dosage ranged from 45 to 110 mg/day. The results of this pilot study showed that amitriptyline is a promising drug for the treatment of prepubertal depression. The patients showed a decrease of dysphoric mood and an increased level of interests, as reflected in increased involvement with other children and playful activities. Serious side effects were not observed and no changes in EKG or blood pressure could be attributed to amitriptyline. A hypomanic reaction developed in an 11-year old boy whose mother had a bipolar disorder and whose father was alcoholic. This "switch phenomenon" suggests that the child may be at risk for the later spontaneous emergence of manic episodes.

Disorders of sleep. Pesikoff and Davis (1971) treated 7 children (6 males, 1 female) ages 19 months to 10.5 years with pavor nocturnus (n = 4), somnambulism (n = 2), or both (n = 1) with imipramine in an open trial. Imipramine dosage ranged from 10 mg to 50 mg at bedtime depending on the weight of the child. All children received medication for a minimum of eight weeks; evaluations were performed monthly. All 7 children's sleep disorders ceased completely. The mechanism of action of imipramine in these cases is unknown; it cannot be explained by a reduction in amount of Stage 4 sleep (imipramine does not significantly alter the quantity of Stage 4 sleep).

Effect on Cognition

There have been only a few studies that included an examination of imipramine's short- or long-term effects on cognition. In general, imipramine was shown to have few, if any, adverse effects on cognitive processes. In two studies (Waizer et al., 1974; Werry et al., 1980) there was the suggestion that imipramine inhibited impulsive responding and increased reflective thought on two different cognitive tasks.

In an outpatient study of six weeks duration, imipramine (mean dose 80 mg/day) was shown to have little, if any, salutary effect on the cognitive performance of 29 hyperactive boys (Rapoport et al., 1974).

In an eight-week outpatient trial (Waizer et al., 1974), 19 hyperkinetic boys (ages 6 to 12 years) received imipramine (mean dose 173.7 mg/day). While receiving imipramine, the children showed less interference with their ability to read correctly the name of a color presented as a discordant "color-word" (Stroop Color-Word Test). This diminished interference could reflect a diminution of impulsivity and a greater ability to pause and reflect prior to responding. The interference measures on this test failed to deteriorate when children were switched to placebo. This could indicate a practice effect due to multiple test administrations and/or sustained improvement after imipramine treatment. Also, there was some minor, although statistically significant, impairment of ability to recall digits in the forward direction.

Thirty hyperactive children received at least a three-week trial of imipramine at a dosage of either 1 or 2 mg/kg/day (Werry et al., 1980). At the end of the trial, they were tested on several cognitive tasks. Although the short-term memory task proved too easy for this sample, significant drug effects were shown for the continuous performance task, a vigilance task reflecting attention span. On the continuous performance task, imipramine significantly reduced the number of commission errors, a reflection of impulsivity. Thus children receiving imipramine were less likely to report erroneously the presence of a stimulus in the absence of its actual presentation. Imipramine did not influence the rating of items on a self-image scale significantly.

Eighteen hyperactive boys were maintained on a mean imipramine dosage of 65.4 mg/day for one year. In these boys, no adverse effects of long-term imipramine treatment on cognitive or intellectual functioning were detected (Quinn & Rapoport, 1975).

IMMEDIATE AND LONG-TERM UNTOWARD EFFECTS

In addition to cardiotoxicity, which will be reviewed in greater detail, and seizures, the major short-term side effects of imipramine can be grouped into three broad categories: autonomic, behavioral, and allergic.

The autonomic side effects are largely due to the relatively high degree of competitive imipramine binding to muscarinic and adrenergic receptors, as well as blockade of biogenic amine reuptake. Autonomic side effects include dry mouth, anorexia, weight loss, nausea, constipation, dizziness, insomnia, drowsiness, increased heart rate, and increased diastolic blood pressure. Frequently, these side effects are transient and disappear with dosage reduction. Behaviorally, transient or dose-dependent irritability, agitation, or worsening of psychosis can emerge. Probable allergic phenomena include worsening of eczema (between fourth and eighth week of treatment) and development of thrombocytopenia (after six months on imipramine).

Seizures and the lowering of the seizure threshold should be recognized as a potential side effect of imipramine therapy. Seizures were reported to occur in three hyperactive/aggressive children, a retarded enuretic child, and an autistic child receiving imipramine therapy (Brown et al., 1973; Petti & Campbell, 1975; Valentine & Maxwell, 1968). Imipramine-induced worsening of preexisting EEG abnormalities, such as increase in spike discharges, occurred in a sample of retarded children without epilepsy (Kajitani, 1963).

Electrocardiographic changes have also been reported during imipramine therapy. Twelve-lead EKGs were obtained on seven severely hyperactive/aggressive children treated with 5 mg/kg/day of imipramine; steady-state plasma levels ranged from 140 to 440 ng/ml (Winsberg et al., 1975). All children showed changes in ventricular repolarization characterized by a decrease in T-wave magnitude and an increase in T-wave width. Three children showed sufficient lengthening of their PR intervals to satisfy criteria for a first-degree atrioventricular block. The heart rate of one child, whose steady-state plasma imipramine level was the lowest (140 ng/ml), rose at least 35 beats/min from baseline to 145/min at steady-state. There was no relationship between the presence of first-degree heart block and steady-state plasma levels.

The cardiotoxic effects of imipramine on the EKGs of 33 children were studied; dosages ranged from 25 to 300 mg/day (Saraf et al., 1978). Treatment resulted in significant increases of heart rate ($p < .0001$) and PR interval ($p < .0001$). In 7 children, the rate-corrected prolongation of the PR interval was above the normal range. An increased PR interval was more likely to occur at a dose of 3.5 mg/kg/day or greater and in children with a shorter pretreatment PR interval. Significant widening of the QRS complex occurred in 3 children; in 1 child, widening occurred on a dosage below 5 mg/kg/day (2.8 mg/kg/day). These EKG changes were detected in the absence of clinical symptomatology.

In a study involving 22 prepubertal depressed children treated with a fixed 75-mg h.s. dose of imipramine, there was no relationship between subjective reports of side effects and plasma concentrations of imipramine and/or desipramine (Preskorn et al., 1983). When the 22 children were stratified according to plasma total tricyclic concentrations, the 6 children whose levels were above 225 ng/ml showed electrocardiographic evidence of slowed cardiac conduction, and increased diastolic blood pressure and heart rate. In 3 children with levels above 350 ng/ml, widening of the PR interval satisfied criteria for first-degree heart block. A confusional state with EEG abnormalities emerged in one child with a plasma total tricyclic level of 481 ng/ml. In the absence of subjective reports of side effects, dosages could be maintained at or raised to dangerously high levels in nonresponders.

Withdrawal emergent symptoms associated with both abrupt and gradual discontinuation of high dosage imipramine therapy in children have been described (Law et al., 1981; Petti & Law, 1981). The symptoms include drowsiness, gastrointestinal complaints, nausea, vomiting, headaches, and a variety of behavioral symptoms (social withdrawal, hyperactivity, depression, provocative behaviors, agitation, and difficulty falling asleep). These withdrawal phenomena have been attributed to "cholinergic rebound" and adrenergic activation. Similar withdrawal phenomena occur in adults.

There are few published data on the long-term side effects of imipramine in children. Of 18 children who received imipramine for one year, anorexia was noted in 39 percent and 3 children complained of occasional irritability. Moreover, maintenance of imipramine therapy for one year resulted in a significant loss of percentile points in weight ($p < 0.01$), but no significant change in the rate of growth for height (Quinn & Rapoport, 1975).

5

LITHIUM CARBONATE

INDICATIONS

Lithium carbonate has been studied in children and adolescents with a variety of psychiatric disorders. Nevertheless, the specific indications for lithium administration to children have not yet been established. At the present time, lithium is not recommended for children under 12 years of age, because of lack of sufficient information about its efficacy and safety in this age group (*Physicians' Desk Reference*, 1985).

In adult psychiatric patients, the use of lithium carbonate is approved only for the specific treatment of manic episodes in manic-depressive illness (Bipolar Disorder, Mixed or Bipolar Disorder, Manic; DSM-III, 1980) and as maintenance therapy to prevent or decrease the number and severity of relapses in these patients (Prien, 1979; Schou, 1983). There is some evidence that lithium is also efficacious in the prophylactic treatment of unipolar affective (depressive) illness in adults (Glen et al., 1984; Schou, 1979).

The use of lithium in children and adolescents has been reviewed by Youngerman and Canino (1978), Lena et al. (1978), Lena (1979), Jefferson (1982), and Campbell, Perry et al. (1984). The reports range from uncontrolled, open studies to double-blind placebo-controlled clinical trials. Based on these studies the following tentative conclusions can be drawn:

> *Bipolar disorder, mixed or manic.* Although rare in prepubertal children, these disorders increase markedly in frequency as adolescence progresses. The few published reports consist of very small sample sizes and therefore no conclusions can be drawn.

> *Major depressive episode.* In children with depressive symptoms whose diagnostic criteria were not adequately defined, lithium was reported to be of benefit. Controls were not employed.

Treatment of aggression, especially impulsive aggression accompanied by explosive affect. Two controlled studies (Campbell, Small et al., 1984; Sheard et al., 1976) have shown that lithium carbonate is statistically superior to placebo in reducing target behaviors. Lithium carbonate was equal or superior to haloperidol in reducing and controlling symptoms of explosive aggressiveness; it had fewer untoward effects than haloperidol, and less adverse effects on cognition (Campbell, Small et al., 1984). Therefore, lithium should be considered a viable alternative when standard treatments (for example, neuroleptics) have not been effective. More research is needed, however, before it can be recommended as the drug of choice.

Mental retardation with symptoms of aggressiveness directed against self and/or others. There is some evidence that lithium may be helpful in decreasing aggressiveness in the mentally retarded. This is particularly important because of the cognitive dulling often reported when neuroleptics are given in sufficiently high doses to reduce aggressiveness.

Behavioral disorders in offspring of lithium-responding parents; behavioral disorders accompanied by mood swings. Preliminary data in these children are inconclusive.

Attention deficit disorder with hyperactivity (ADDH). Lithium has not proven an efficacious drug in this disorder.

Pervasive developmental disorder: infantile autism. It appears that aggressiveness directed against self or others may be responsive to lithium.

CONTRAINDICATIONS AND INTERACTIONS WITH OTHER DRUGS

Administration of lithium is contraindicated in individuals with a history or evidence of renal, cardiac, or thyroid diseases. It should not be administered to teenagers at risk for pregnancy because of its cardiac teratogenicity, particularly Ebstein's anomaly. Källén and Tanberg (1983) reported that 7 percent of pregnant women who used lithium in early pregnancy delivered infants with serious heart defects; none of the infants, however, had Ebstein's anomaly.

The interactions of lithium and other drugs, including neuroleptics, have been recently reviewed (Jefferson et al., 1981; Reisberg & Gershon, 1979). Clearly, one must be aware of potential drug interactions before prescribing lithium to a patient already receiving other medications. Although the exact causal relationship has not been determined, severe, irreversible brain damage, persistent dyskinesias, and the neuroleptic malignant syndrome have been reported in adults to whom lithium and neuroleptics (haloperidol and thioridazine) have been administered in high doses simultaneously (Cohen & Cohen, 1974; Spring & Frankel, 1981). On the other hand, many patients have received haloperidol and lithium together with no adverse effects.

DOSAGE

The lithium ion is usually administered orally as lithium carbonate (Li_2CO_3), a highly soluble salt (lithium citrate syrup is also available). Complete absorption occurs in approximately 8 hours and peak plasma concentrations occur within 2 to 4 hours (Baldessarini, 1980). About 95 percent of a single dose of lithium is excreted in the urine, between one-third and two-thirds within 6 to 12 hours, and the remainder over the next 10 to 14 days. This same excretion pattern occurs after cessation of lithium therapy (Baldessarini, 1980). Because of the pharmacokinetic profile and the low therapeutic index of the lithium ion, immediate-release capsules or tablets must be given in divided doses, usually three or four times daily to avoid toxicity. Controlled-release Li_2CO_3 tablets are available and are administered twice daily.

Steady-state concentrations of lithium usually occur 5 to 6 days after repeated identical daily doses. Baldessarini and Stephens (1970) have noted that lithium pharmacokinetics differ considerably among individuals, but they are fairly stable over time in the same individual. Serum lithium levels should be determined when lithium concentrations are relatively stable, for example, 12 hours after the previous dose, and immediately before the morning dose.

Lithium toxicity is closely related to serum lithium levels. Toxicity may occur close to therapeutic serum levels, so administration should be carried out only when prompt and accurate serum lithium measurements are readily available. Also, because lithium decreases sodium reuptake by the renal tubules, it is important to maintain adequate sodium (salt) and fluid intake. In summer, children and adolescents can be particularly susceptible to dehydration secondary to excessive perspiration, and serum levels of lithium may become elevated to toxic levels despite constant dosage.

Therapeutic dosages of lithium in older children and adolescents do not differ from those in adults (Campbell, Perry et al., 1984). Serum lithium levels between 0.6 and 1.2 mEq/1 are recommended for long-term maintenance. This can usually be achieved by administration of lithium in divided total daily doses of 900 to 1200 mg.

The lithium starting dosage should be low, perferably 300 mg daily with gradual increments. Dosage must be individually titrated according to both serum lithium levels and clinical response. During active regulation, twice weekly monitoring of lithium levels is recommended (Campbell, Perry et al., 1984). Lithium levels in saliva are about 2.5 times greater than in serum, as shown in Figure 6, and may be used to monitor lithium (Perry et al., 1984; Shopsin et al., 1969). However, periodic serum checks are still needed at fixed intervals.

Dosage should be gradually increased until therapeutic serum levels or remission of symptoms occurs or untoward effects prevent further increase. Some early side effects (nausea, diarrhea, muscle weakness, thirst, urinary frequency, hand tremor, and a dazed feeling) are related to too rapid a rise and to peaks in serum lithium levels (Schou, 1969; Sheard, 1975). In most cases, they can be avoided by a low initial daily dose of lithium given in divided doses after meals, and gradual increments of dosage. When these side effects occur, they will usually spontaneously subside within a few days.

Compliance

Sheard (1975) has called particular attention to the relationship between untoward effects and drug compliance. He noted that individuals being treated for aggressive behavioral disorders seem to tolerate side effects poorly and cautions that side effects may be used by them as an excuse to discontinue treatment.

SHORT- AND LONG-TERM EFFICACY

Short-Term Effect on Behavioral Symptoms

Lithium administration has resulted in clinical improvement in some children and adolescents who had mood disturbance, especially manic-depressive illness; cyclic mood swings; or behavioral disturbances with explosiveness and aggressiveness.

There are several reports in the literature of children and adolescents diagnosed with manic-depressive illness (or a synonym thereof) who benefited from lithium carbonate (Berg et al., 1974; Brumback &

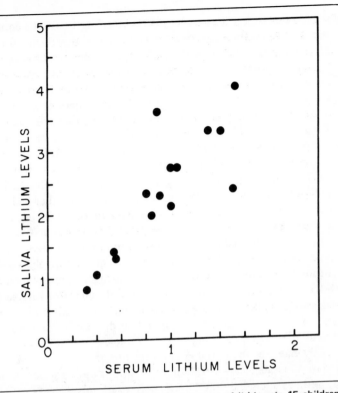

Figure 6: Saliva and serum levels on optimal dosages of lithium in 15 children ages 6.0 to 11.3 years with undersocialized, aggressive conduct disorder. (From Perry et al., 1984, *Journal of Clinical Psychopharmacology*; reprinted with permission.)

Weinberg, 1977; Carlson & Strober, 1978; Feinstein & Wolpert, 1973; Horowitz, 1977; Kelley et al., 1976; McKnew et al., 1981; Van der Velde, 1970; Warneke, 1975; White & O'Shanick, 1977; Youngerman & Canino, 1983).

DeLong (1978) reported on 12 children, mean age 9.5 years (range 4 to 14 years), with severe chronic behavior disorders including hostility, explosive anger, aggressiveness, and distractibility. Nine had cyclic extreme mood swings suggestive of manic-depressive illness. Family histories were strongly positive for manic-depressive disease, depression, and alcoholism. Dosage of lithium carbonate ranged from 450 to

1200 mg/day (serum lithium level 0.5 to 1.2 mEq/1). All 12 children were maintained on lithium for a mean of 18 months (range 6 to 33 months). According to the author, all responded with a striking improvement in mood that seemed fundamental to the overall improvement. The hostility, anger, and aggressive outbursts improved consistently and the cyclic behavioral extremes were attenuated or ceased. Academic performance increased notably in five. This study had several methodological problems. DeLong's 12 subjects were selected from a larger group of 40 children based on their beneficial responses to lithium over a period of at least 6 months. The children were diagnostically heterogeneous. Only 4 children were evaluated using a double-blind placebo-controlled crossover design; the other 8 children had uncontrolled trials of discontinuing lithium and reducing dosage during treatment. DeLong et al.'s subsequent (1983) study was a double-blind placebo-controlled crossover discontinuation study of lithium's effects on specific behaviors in 11 children who had putatively benefited from lithium. Diagnostic criteria were more stringent and included most DSM-III criteria for mania. Many of these children (11 of 16) had been treated with stimulants for an attention deficit; although these children benefited from lithium, the attention deficit did not improve substantially. The diagnostic meaning of this is unclear. Most children have previously had an open trial of lithium discontinuation and it was elected to reinstate treatment. Other limitations of this study, as noted by the authors, included that the trial periods of only 3 weeks may have been too short to elicit the full effect of treatment changes, and the small number of children.

Hassanyeh and Davison (1980) reported on ten cases of bipolar affective psychosis (5 males and 5 females) with onset before 16 years of age (mean 14.1 years). Seven of these patients eventually received lithium. At the time of lithium administration their ages ranged from 13 to 18 years. Lithium was efficacious in six; serum levels from 0.6 to 1.0 mEq/1 were maintained for from 6 months to 5 years (mean 3 years). The seven lithium-treated patients tended to have shorter episodes of illness and significantly shorter depressive episodes ($p < 0.05$) than the three patients not treated with lithium. There was no difference in the number of episodes of illness between the two groups.

Frommer (1968) and Annell (1969a, 1969b) used lithium to treat a total of 36 children who had depressive features. The samples seemed to be diagnostically heterogeneous; the studies were uncontrolled; and many of the children received amitryptyline concurrently. Frommer

(1968) used very low doses (50-250 mg/day) and therapeutic serum levels may not have been reached. McKnew et al. (1981) reported that 2 boys with DSM-III major depressive disorder failed to respond to lithium in a double-blind placebo-controlled crossover design.

Sheard's (1975) review of animal and human data is recommended for background on the antiaggressive effects of lithium. Sheard (1975) administered lithium carbonate to 12 adolescent males in a correctional facility who had habitual impulsive and aggressive behavior. During incarceration and following release, the number of serious (violent) aggressive episodes decreased markedly when serum levels were increased at least 0.6 mEq/l compared to lower values (10 versus 26 incidents). Total number of all antisocial incidents was less prominently affected (64 versus 89 incidents).

Sheard et al. (1976) conducted a well-designed placebo-controlled, double-blind study of the effect of lithium carbonate on chronic impulsive aggressive behavior. Subjects were 66 nonpsychotic prisoners aged 16 to 24 years old; 34 subjects received lithium (20 for three months, 8 for two months, and 6 for one month). Similar numbers received placebo. Over the period of study the mean lithium carbonate doses ranged from 1212 mg/day to 1691 mg/day, with serum lithium values of 0.64 to 0.89 mEq/l. The lithium group had significantly fewer major and total number of infractions than the placebo group.

Siassi (1982) conducted a study of 14 boys ages 7 to 13 years who were unmanageable in the community, displayed sporadic unprovoked physical aggression, and were refractory to usual treatments. They were matched with boys in the school with similar characteristics but without undue aggressiveness. During a three-month pretreatment rating period, the experimental group had significantly more unprovoked aggressive acts (14.8 versus 1.8, $p < .01$). The aggressive youngsters were maintained on lithium carbonate, mean dose 1475 mg/day (range 900-2100 mg/day) and mean serum level 1.21 mEq/l (range 1.01 to 1.43 mEq/l). The number of aggressive acts by the experimental group declined dramatically to 3.9 and was not significantly different from the nonaggressive controls that remained at 1.8. During three post-treatment months, following the discontinuation of lithium, the behavior of the experimental group deteriorated and again became significantly worse than controls (11.9 versus 1.7, $p < .01$). The authors noted that none of the children showed typical mania or depression.

Campbell, Anderson, Cohen et al. (1982) assigned 15 aggressive hospitalized male children in a double-blind pilot study to lithium carbonate, haloperidol, or chlorpromazine. The diagnoses of the 5 children receiving lithium were unsocialized aggressive (3), schizophrenia (1), infantile autism (1); their ages ranged from 6 years, 3 months to 11 years, 9 months. The mean optimal dose of lithium carbonate was 1800 mg/day (range 1250 to 2000 mg/day; serum lithium range 0.76 to 1.24 mEq/1, saliva range 1.25 to 2.10 mEq/1). Lithium, haloperidol, and chlorpromazine were all equally effective in reducing angry affect, bullying, distractibility, fighting, hyperactivity, negativism, and temper tantrums; however, chlorpromazine was excessively sedating at relatively low doses. The encouraging results in this study led to a double-blind, placebo-controlled study in which the behavioral efficacy of haloperidol and lithium carbonate were compared in 61 hospitalized children aged 5.2 to 12.9 years diagnosed as conduct disorder, undersocialized aggressive type according to DSM-III (1980) criteria (Campbell, Small et al., 1984). These children exhibited a behavioral profile of severe aggressiveness, explosiveness, and disruptiveness unresponsive to various outpatient treatments, including pharmacotherapy. They had had no evidence of psychosis, mental retardation or clinical seizure disorder. There were 82 children enrolled in this clinical trial; 21 dropped out during the two-week placebo baseline period, over three-fourths because the symptoms of severe aggressiveness and explosiveness ameliorated to such an extent over the two-week period that they did not require medication. The remaining children were assigned randomly to haloperidol (N = 20), lithium carbonate (N = 21), or placebo (N = 20) for four weeks of treatment. Dose was regulated by incremental steps during the first two weeks and the children continued on their optimal doses for the final two weeks. During dosage regulation, saliva was collected twice weekly in all children to maintain blind experimental conditions and serum lithium levels were determined at termination of the study for those children receiving lithium. Optimal doses of lithium carbonate ranged from 500 to 2000 mg/day (mean 1166 mg/day). For these doses, the saliva lithium level ranged from 0.32 to 1.51 mEq/1 (mean 0.993 mEq/1). For lithium, higher optimal doses correlated with increasing age and weight.

Both lithium carbonate and haloperidol were significantly superior to placebo in reducing target behaviors on a number of rating scales, specifically angry affect, bullying, distractibility, fighting, hyperactivity, negativism, and temper tantrums. A rating by ward staff of clinical improvement on optimal dosage before the code was broken turned out to be highly significant ($p < .00005$). None of the children was depressed as assessed by history, clinical examination, or on the CPRS. Patients receiving lithium experienced fewer untoward effects than those on haloperidol, although this did not reach significance. Importantly, child psychiatrists rated the untoward effects in children on optimal doses of lithium as interfering less with the child's daily functioning than those of haloperidol. Clinically, staff felt that lithium's primary action was to decrease the explosive affect, and that other behavioral improvements were secondary to this; haloperidol, however, merely made the child more manageable. No child had a history of manic-depressive illness in his or her family, but several of the parents, especially in the lithium group, had histories of depression, alcoholism, or drug abuse.

Behaviorally disordered children of lithium-responding parents. Three studies (Dyson & Barcai, 1970; McKnew et al., 1981; and Youngerman & Canino, 1983) have specifically looked at a total of 9 children with behavioral disturbances whose parents were known lithium responders. Of 9 children, 5 improved, but 2 of the 5 were themselves manic-depressives, so the efficacy in this group of children is still unclear.

Treatment of children and adolescents with behavioral disorders accompanied by mood swings. Rifkin et al. (1972) studied 21 subjects, mostly adolescent females, with Emotionally Unstable Character Disorder on a double-blind, random-assignment crossover study comparing six weeks of lithium carbonate with six weeks of placebo. The subjects had chronic maladaptive behavioral patterns consisting of short depressive and manic mood swings, lasting hours to a few days. Usually the episodes were not precipitated by, or reactive to, environmental or interpersonal events. The subjects had difficulty in accepting reasonable authority, in being appropriately self-reliant, and were sometimes overreactive. They often abused drugs, especially amphetamines and marijuana, avoided school or work, malingered, were sexually promiscuous, and engaged in delinquent behavior. Serum lithium levels were maintained between 0.6 and 1.5 mEq/l. Of 21 subjects, 14 were judged better on the Oklahoma Behavior Rating Scale while receiving lithium carbonate, 4 were better on placebo, and 3 showed no difference between the two conditions. The improvement on lithium carbonate was statistically significant ($p < .02$). Mood swings also decreased on lithium.

Lena et al. (1978) reported preliminary data on 5 children who had "episodic mood and behavioral disturbance." Further diagnostic details were not described. They were administered lithium (serum levels 0.7 to 1.2 mEq/1) in a double-blind crossover design with eight weeks on lithium and placebo; 2 children improved markedly, 2 moderately, and 1 equivocally. In 2, behavioral improvements were accompanied by improvement in school performance.

Mental retardation with symptoms of aggressiveness directed against self and/or others. Goetzl et al. (1977) administered lithium carbonate to three cases of mildly to moderately retarded adolescents with severely disruptive behavior characterized by aggressiveness and hyperactivity. Two had reported mood swings. Administration of lithium carbonate resulted in a marked reduction of maladaptive behavior in all three. Maintenance dosage was 1200 mg daily resulting in serum lithium levels of 0.7 to 0.9 mEq/1.

Dale (1980) treated 15 aggressive retarded patients with lithium carbonate; 4 were adolescents (age 17 to 19), 2 males and 2 females. Lithium dosage ranged from 750 to 3000 mg/day (serum range 0.4 to 2.0 mEq/1; average 0.58 mEq/1). Three patients improved, showing a sustained reduction in aggressive behavior, and 1 worsened. Those patients who responded well did so within one to two weeks.

Dostal (1972) administered lithium to 14 severely disturbed retarded adolescent boys who had prolonged outbursts of anger, aggressiveness, and hyperactivity, and had failed to respond to phenothiazines. Of these, 4 were profoundly, 3 severely, 6 moderately, and 1 mildly retarded; 3 had grand mal seizures, and 2 had paralysis of the lower limbs. Lithium was gradually increased over a period of four months to maintain mean serum lithium levels about 0.9 mEq/1 (range 0.7-1.2 mEq/1), and psychoactive medication (other than anticonvulsants) was discontinued after two months. After eight months of lithium there was significant improvement in affect, aggressiveness, psychomotor activity, and restlessness (p < .01), and undisciplined behavior (p < .05). Improvements correlated with serum lithium levels. The incidence of acute outbursts of aggressive behavior decreased by 65 percent during the period on lithium.

The best therapeutic gains occurred in patients with marked excitability and impulsive primitive aggressiveness (biting, destruction of objects, and mutilation "as a non-specific reaction"); in patients with periods of more deteriorated behavioral disturbance alternating with periods of relative calm; and in patients with "marked periodic changes in affectivity or emotional lability." Patients whose hyperkinetic behavior lacked any affective component, but instead was characterized by "spastic irritability," continuous total body restlessness, repeated minor "auto-mutilations," stereotypies, or ritualistic movements showed almost no improvement (Dostal, 1972, p. 496).

Side effects were rather specific for this group of mentally retarded patients. Of especial significance were polydipsia and polyuria. The patients drank any liquid available and had a subsequent enormous polyuria including nocturnal enuresis that alienated caretakers. This ceased within two weeks of discontinuing lithium therapy.

Pervasive developmental disorder: infantile autism. Gram and Rafaelsen (1972) treated 18 children and adolescents ages 8 to 22 years who had psychoses or pronounced psychotic traits from before age five; 9 (5 males, 4 females) had infantile psychosis. Lithium (serum range 0.6-1.0 mEq/l) was administered in a twelve-month long double-blind placebo-controlled design with crossover at six months time; patients were assigned randomly. Patients were rated by teachers and parents and improved significantly on lithium ($p < .05$). The symptoms that most frequently improved were disturbed activity, aggression, depressed or elevated mood, speech disturbances, and stereotypies.

Campbell, Fish, Korein et al. (1972) compared lithium and chlorpromazine in a crossover design involving ten children ages 3 to 6 years, most of whom were autistic. There were no significant differences between drugs or between placebo baseline and treatment. One child, however, showed dramatic relief of severe autoaggression marked by head-banging, biting of his forearms, and violent temper tantrums. He was the only child who had had explosive affect. His optimal dose of lithium carbonate was 600 mg daily (on optimal dose serum lithium levels ranged from 0.59 to 0.76 mEq/l). His gains disappeared following discontinuation of lithium.

Attention deficit disorder with hyperactivity. Lithium was not effective in severe hyperactivity. Nine severely hyperactive children (ages 8 to 14 years) who were unresponsive to dextroamphetamine, methylphenidate, chlorpromazine, diphenhydramine, and diphenylhydantoin failed to respond to lithium carbonate (Greenhill et al., 1973). Whitehead and Clark (1970) also found no significant differences between lithium and placebo in 7 hyperactive children. However, this small sample was diagnostically heterogeneous, and the authors may have used subtherapeutic serum lithium levels. DeLong and Nieman (1983) noted that lithium was not effective in significantly improving short attention span in their study of 16 hyperactive, irritable, excitable, aggressive, and depressed children with symptoms suggesting manic-depressive illness.

Long-Term Effect on Behavioral Symptoms

Hassanyeh and Davison (1980, reviewed above) gave six bipolar patients lithium for up to five years. They reported that long-term side effects were not a serious problem in these six patients. In analyzing long-term efficacy, the authors included a seventh patient whose lithium was discontinued after one month because of nausea and vomiting. Depressive episodes were significantly shorter in these seven patients compared to three non-lithium-treated patients (p < 0.05). Although there was no significant difference in the number of episodes of illness between the two groups, those on lithium showed a tendency to have shorter episodes of illness.

DeLong (1978) treated patients for up to 33 months. He noted a decrease in effectiveness of lithium in a few children, but in the majority there was no loss of efficacy. Dale (1980) treated some retarded adolescents for up to five years. Kelly et al. (1976) treated adolescents for four years, and Horowitz (1977) for over two years, with good control of symptoms.

Self-mutilating behavior of 11 years duration, which had resulted in bone deformities and scars, ceased completely and remained in remission in an autistic child throughout more than five years of maintenance on lithium (B. Shopsin, personal communication).

Effects of Lithium on Cognition

Platt et al. (1984) have reviewed the effects of lithium on cognition in adults; at present only two studies involving children have been published (Greenhill et al., 1973; Platt et al., 1984).

In a sample of nine hyperactive children, there were no significant differences between lithium and placebo in reaction time with either long or short preparatory time; it is not clear how many of the nine children showed improvement in the long preparatory interval reaction time (Greenhill et al., 1973).

Platt et al. (1984) reported on the cognitive effects of lithium carbonate on 21 children, after four weeks maintenance at an average dose of 1166 mg/day, (range 500-2000 mg/day). Serum levels averaged 0.933 mEq/1 (range 0.32-1.51 mEq/1). These subjects were a subset of 61 treatment-resistant children, ages 5.2 to 12.9 years, who were hospitalized; their mean IQ was 87.6. They were randomly assigned to lithium, haloperidol, or placebo (Campbell, Small et al., 1984). A cognitive battery was administered on baseline and at the end of treatment. It consisted of six components chosen to assess various aspects of cognition: Reaction Time (RT) Task, Porteus Maze Test, Matching Familiar Figures (MFF) Test, Short-Term Recognition Memory (STRM) Test, Concept Attainment Task, and the Stroop Test, which measures the ability to inhibit a dominant response when two responses compete. The main effect of lithium was on the Porteus Maze qualitative scores which measure motor performance, the ability or willingness to follow directions, and the neatness and control of the performance. The children receiving lithium had significantly higher scores—indicating poorer performance—than children who received haloperidol or placebo. The Porteus Maze test quotient, which assesses nonverbal intelligence, did not change from baseline to the end of the four-week treatment period for the lithium group; however, 3 of the children showed large improvements and 5 showed large decrements. There were no significant effects of lithium carbonate on any of the other tasks.

To date, there are no studies of long-term cognitive effects of lithium carbonate.

UNTOWARD EFFECTS

Mild to Moderate Untoward Effects

Both short- and long-term untoward effects have been recently reviewed (Jenner, 1979; Lydiard & Gelenberg, 1982; Reisberg & Gershon, 1979). Early-onset side effects of lithium carbonate administration are nausea, diarrhea, muscle weakness, thirst, urinary frequency, a dazed feeling, and hand tremor. These side effects seem to be related to the amount and absorption rate of lithium entering the circulation (Schou, 1969; Sheard, 1975). Among the later onset side effects, Sheard (1975) noted a continued hand tremor (unresponsive to antiparkinsonian drugs), polydipsia, polyuria, or a vasopressin-resistant diabetes insipidus which requires cessation of treatment.

Relatively few reports record careful observations of side effects in relation to lithium dosages and serum levels in children and adolescents. There is some evidence that untoward effects may be somewhat different in children (Campbell, Perry et al., 1984) and may vary according to diagnosis (Dostal, 1972). Although the *Physicians' Desk Reference* (1985) states that adverse reactions to lithium seldom occur at serum levels below 1.5 mEq/l, except in occasional patients sensitive to lithium, we have not found this to be the case in our work with children (Campbell, Anderson, Cohen et al., 1982; Campbell, Cohen et al., 1982; Campbell, Fish, Korein et al., 1972; Campbell, Small et al., 1984). Untoward effects have frequently occurred at serum levels well below 1.5 mEq/l as shown in Table 5 (Campbell, Perry et al., 1984). The most common untoward effects observed in these 36 children aged 3 to 13 years—of whom 24 were diagnosed as undersocialized aggressive conduct disorders, 8 infantile autism, and 4 other diagnoses—were weight gain, excessive sedation, decreased motor activity, irritability, stomach ache, vomiting, tremor, pallor, and headache. Some of these untoward effects were noted on as little as 250 mg/day and with serum lithium levels as low as 0.3 mEq/l. Two five-year olds developed reversible EKG changes on daily doses of 900 mg lithium carbonate. One had a mild right ventricular conduction delay with serum lithium levels of 0.575 mEq/l and the other a sinus arrhythmia (possibly an atrioventricular nodal rhythm) with a serum lithium level of 1.025 mEq/l. Campbell, Fish, Korein et al. (1972) noted decreased thyroxine iodine in two children.

Lithium Toxicity

Lithium toxicity is closely related to serum lithium levels and there is a relatively narrow margin between therapeutic and toxic levels. The likelihood of toxicity increases with increasing serum levels and mild to moderate toxic reactions may occur at levels from 1.5 to 2.5 mEq/l and moderate to severe reactions may occur at levels from 2.0 to 2.5 mEq/l. Onset is usually gradual and primarily affects the nervous system. Indeed, behavioral toxicity may be the earliest sign of lithium intoxication. Poisoning from toxic levels is usually an exaggeration of the early side effects with additional muscle hyperirritability, sluggishness, slurred speech, ataxia, anorexia, stupor, coma, and death. No specific antidote for lithium poisoning is known, so careful monitoring and early recognition and management of dehydration, electrolyte imbalance, and infection are essential.

TABLE 5   Short-Term Untoward Effects of Lithium Carbonate
in 36 Children[a]

Untoward Effects (number of patients)	Dosage Range (mg/day)	Serum Level (mEq/l)	Saliva Level (mEq/l)
Weight gain (16)	500-2000	0.30-1.53	1.00-5.05
Weight loss (5)	500-1250	1.01-1.50	1.59-3.36
Decreased appetite (4)	500-900	0.8-1.225	2.01
Stomachache (7)	250-1750	—	1.372-2.93
Nausea (3)	750-1500	—	2.87-3.65
Vomiting (7)	450-1500	0.450-1.275	4.01
Diarrhea/loose bowel movements (4)	600-1350	0.550-1.483	—
Polydipsia (3)	450-1350	0.375-2.075	—
Urinary frequency/ Polyuria (4)	600-900	0.475-1.160	—
Diurnal enuresis (1)	600	—	—
Headache (6)	500-1750	—	1.34-3.65
Dizziness (2)	1250-1350	—	2.21
Pallor (6)	450-1500	0.45-1.16	1.75
Decreased verbal production (1)	750	—	1.68
Dysarthria, slurred speech (5)	450-1350	0.6	1.25
Tearful (1)	500-750	—	1.11-1.68
Irritability (7)	450-1350	0.45-1.09	—
Fatigue/lethargy (4)	750-1750	1.15	2.05-2.16
Subdued (1)	750	—	1.68
"Glazed look"/as if in a daze (5)	450-1500	0.91	—
Decreased motor activity (9)	450-1750	0.91-1.46	—
Feeling "tired and miserable" or "sick" (3)	450-1350	0.325-1.460	—
Excessive sedation (10)	750-2000	0.95-2.075	1.88-2.05
Insomnia (2)	1300-2000	0.91	—
Fidgetiness (1)	1250	—	2.21
Motor excitation (5)	450-900	0.111	—
Tremor (7)	1250-1500	—	1.88-3.65
Ataxia (5)	1250-1350	—	1.25
Drooling (1)	1350	1.95	—
Achy lower extremities (1)	1350	1.46	—
EKG changes (2)[b]	900	—	—

(continued)

TABLE 5 Continued

Untoward Effects (number of patients)	Dosage Range (mg/day)	Serum Level (mEq/1)	Saliva Level (mEq/1)
Leukocytosis with lymphocytopenia (4)	600-1350	0.30-0.95	—
Decrease of T_4 (2)	600-900	0.55-1.05	—
Worsening of psychosis (3)[c]	600-900	1.16	—
Toxic confusional state moderate (1)[d]	1750	2.85	—
Worsening of EEG (12)[e]	500-2000	0.32-1.51	0.81-5.05

SOURCE: Reproduced with permission of *Psychosomatics*; from Campbell, Perry, & Green (1984).

a. Children were ages 3 to 13 years; conduct disorder, unsocialized, aggressive, N = 24; infantile autism, N = 8; other, N = 4. (From Campbell, Fish, David et al., 1972; Campbell, Anderson, Small et al., 1982; Campbell, Anderson, Deutsch et al., 1984.
b. EKGs were done only in 10 subjects (Campbell, Fish, David et al., 1972).
c. Only 9 of 36 subjects were psychotic.
d. This was above optimal dose and secondary to dehydration in summer.
e. EEGs were done in 17 subjects (Bennett et al., 1983).

EEG and Lithium Administration in Children

Bennett et al. (1983) reported on the EEGs of 17 children ages 5.2 to 12.9 years who received lithium carbonate. These children all had conduct disorder and were part of a larger study (Campbell, Small et al., 1984). On baseline four children had normal EEGs and 13 had abnormal EEGs. Following four weeks on lithium 500 mg to 2000 mg/day (mean 1250 mg/day) with serum levels of 0.32 to 1.51 mEq/day (mean 1.03), 3 EEGs were normal and 14 were abnormal. Of particular interest, however, was the fact that 12 of the EEGs worsened, whereas 4 were different or better and 1 remained the same. This was statistically different from the EEG changes of children on placebo (p < 0.001) where only 3 worsened. However, it was not statistically different from the group of 15 children who received haloperidol, 8 of whose EEGs worsened on drug.

The EEG changes associated with lithium are sufficiently characteristic so that a trained electroencephalographer can identify by EEG alone children treated with lithium, haloperidol, or placebo (Bennett et al., 1983). Although the worsening of EEG in these children is a marker of toxicity, the changes on the EEG were more abnormal than one might predict from the children's behavior, and there was no correlation between degree of EEG worsening and clinical toxicity. This may be different from adults where clinical change on lithium carbonate is not related to EEG changes and in whom the presence and severity of EEG change is correlated with neurotoxicity (Johnson et al., 1970).

Although the EEG may prove more useful as a sensitive monitor of toxic changes secondary to lithium carbonate than clinically observable signs or behaviors, proof of this will require large numbers of subjects. As a practical matter, EEG worsening as indicated by paroxysmal features, such as spikes, spikes and waves, focal slow delta waves, and/or severe diffuse slowing (e.g., slowing of alpha-waves to 7 cps), should alert the clinician to monitor the EEG regularly. EEGS should be recorded on the same day as serum lithium levels are determined to faciliate correlation.

Lithium and the Kidney

Renal biopsy studies have found a higher than expected incidence of interstitial fibrosis in the kidneys of adult lithium patients. Despite the presence of this nonspecific morphological damage to the kidney, renal function appears to be well preserved even in patients who have been taking lithium for many years (Schou & Vestergaard, 1981). Renal failure appears to be extremely rare. Nevertheless, routine monitoring of renal function is recommended. Clinicians differ on the extent of this monitoring. Jefferson et al. (1983) measure serum creatinine every six months. Some clinicians advocate more aggressive monitoring of renal function, consisting of 24-hour urine volume, creatinine clearance, urinalysis, and a renal concentration test, such as the response to extrinsic vasopressin. In view of the absence of any long-term studies of lithium administration to children, potential renal hazards remain unknown and renal functioning must be monitored periodically. For a review, Jenner's article (1977) is recommended.

6

✓ BENZODIAZEPINES

INDICATIONS

Little is known about the safety and efficacy of benzodiazepines in psychiatric disorders of children and adolescents. In younger children these drugs are prescribed primarily for anticonvulsant activity and the management of disorders of sleep. Prescribing patterns for adolescents are similar to those for adults (Coffey et al., 1983).

The use of benzodiazepines in child psychiatry has been reviewed by Greenblatt and Shader (1974), Rapoport et al. (1978b), and Petti (in press). The published reports on the use of the benzodiazepines—particularly well-designed placebo-controlled studies—are few. The following preliminary and tentative conclusions may be drawn from the available literature, and from our clinical experience.

Sleep disorders. Rapoport, Mikkelsen et al. (1978) note that acute sleep disturbances such as insomnia and night waking may be interrupted by a short course of treatment with a short-acting benzodiazepine. The benzodiazepines decrease the amount of stage IV sleep in virtually all published sleep studies (Greenblatt & Shader, 1974); theoretically, they should be useful in treating night terrors (pavor nocturnus) and somnambulism (sleepwalking). Glick et al. (1971) used diazepam to treat seven children aged 7 to 11 years; three had somnambulism and pavor nocturnus; the others had insomnia. Diazepam (2 to 5 mg) was administered within one hour of bedtime. All seven patients responded favorably.

Preanaesthesia. Gittleman-Klein (1978) noted that the benzodiazepines are useful preanaesthetic agents for children and adolescents, because they may reduce situational and anticipatory anxiety.

Neurotic anxiety. An open study of 51 diagnostically heterogeneous children with anxiety found that about two-thirds, especially children with adjustment reaction, improved on chlordiazepoxide (Krakowski, 1963). Lucas and Pasley (1969) found little clinically apparent benefit from diazepam in a double-blind placebo-controlled study of 12 children and adolescents with anxiety and acting-out behavior.

Behavioral disorders. Kraft et al. (1965) administered chlordiazepoxide to 130 children with various behavioral disorders; 41 percent improved. Similarly, Breitner (1962) found that daily doses of 20 to 50 mg of the drug were useful in treating juvenile delinquents and making them more accessible for psychotherapy. Although Gleser et al. (1965) also found a positive effect of chlordiazepoxide in delinquents, theirs was an acute single-dose experiment and does not reveal much about the short- or long-term efficacy in this patient population.

School phobia. There is some suggestion that the benzodiazepines in small doses decrease anxiety in these children and mobilize them to return to school (D'Amato, 1962; Klein et al., 1980; Kraft et al., 1965).

Mental retardation with behavior disorder. Chlordiazepoxide worsened target symptoms, although not significantly, in the only double-blind study involving retarded children and adolescents (LaVeck & Buckey, 1961). In two open studies, about half the patients improved whereas about one-fourth remained unchanged and the other fourth became worse (Krakowski, 1963; Pilkington, 1961).

Depression. Frommer (1967, p. 731) claimed that chlordiazepoxide was a useful adjunct to antidepressants in treating depressed children. She noted that "its tranquilizing and disinhibiting effects offer early relief from the tension and anxiety which are part of the depressive picture in so many." The difficulty in distinguishing the relative therapeutic effects of antidepressants and chlordiazepoxide, and the apparent diagnostic heterogeneity of Frommer's sample, make the results of this study difficult to interpret.

Enuresis. Kline (1968) administered diazepam or placebo to 50 children and adolescents age 3 to 15 with nocturnal enuresis in a double-blind study. Organic uropathy and mental retardation were exclusion criteria. Initially, diazepam was given in a dose of 5 mg in the morning and 10 mg at night. This was increased to a maximum of 25 mg if no positive response occurred at a lower dosage. After the code was broken, it was determined that the 28 children who received diazepam were significantly improved after 4 weeks ($p < .05$), compared to the 22 who received placebo.

Specific developmental disorder: severe reading retardation. As reviewed under Stimulants, Aman and Werry (1982) compared the effects of diazepam to those of methylphenidate in 15 children. They concluded that neither drug was useful in these children.

Hyperkinetic syndrome (ADDH). The benzodiazepines are not indicated in the treatment of Attention Deficit Disorder with Hyperactivity (hyperkinetic syndrome). Zrull et al. (1963) found that both chlordiazepoxide and d-amphetamine were more effective than placebo, but d-amphetamine tended to be more effective than chlordiazepoxide. Zrull et al. (1964) compared diazepam, d-amphetamine, and placebo in treating 21 hyperkinetic children (19 boys, 2 girls) ages 6 to 12 years, who showed hyperactivity, distractibility, impulsivity, and emotional instability. Again, d-amphetamine was best. Diazepam was worse than placebo. Although Zrull and colleagues (1963, 1964) state that their patients were suffering from hyperkinetic syndrome, it is apparent that they were diagnostically heterogeneous and included diagnoses of anxiety neurosis, organic brain syndrome, and borderline psychosis.

Schizophrenia. The few child or adolescent schizophrenics who were tested on benzodiazepines responded with a worsening of psychosis (Lucas & Pasley, 1969; Petti et al., 1982; Pilkington, 1961).

Contraindications. Benzodiazepines are contraindicated in the presence of acute narrow-angle glaucoma. They are *relatively* contraindicated in addiction-prone individuals. Finally, the use of benzodiazepines during the first trimester of pregnancy has been related to fetal malformations.

DOSAGE

The benzodiazepines are prescribed for the relief of anxiety, sedation, and induction of sleep. They are also used as anticonvulsants and as muscle relaxants. A benzodiazepine should be selected for its speed of action and effective half-life, which is a function of both metabolism and elimination. Dosage of a specific drug depends upon the therapuetic effect that is desired, such as anxiety reduction or sedation. Baldessarini (1980) has pointed out that there exist marked differences in absorption rates among the various benzodiazepines; for example, peak plasma levels of diazepam may be reached in about an hour in adults although peak levels of chlordiazepoxide may not be reached for several hours. He also notes that diazepam is more quickly absorbed in children and peak serum levels may be reached in only 15 to 30 minutes. Coffey et al. (1983) have reviewed the pharmacokinetics of the benzodiazepines and shown that their metabolism is different for children and adults, at least in some cases.

Diazepam and chlordiazepoxide are the only benzodiazepines that have been used frequently in children.

Because antianxiety effects, sedation, and psychomotor impairment can occur at about the same blood concentrations (Baldessarini, 1980) when the lessening of anxiety is the primary goal, a benzodiazpine should be administered in divided doses to avoid excessive sedation.

Other uses of the benzodiazepines, such as for relief of spasticity, cerebral palsy, preanaesthesia medication, or as an anticonvulsant, will not be discussed here. For a discussion of tolerance, addiction, and the withdrawal syndrome, the adult addiction literature is recommended.

SHORT- AND LONG-TERM EFFICACY

Effect on Behavioral Symptoms

In an open study, Krakowski (1963) administered chlordiazepoxide to 51 subjects, ages 4 to 16 years, who were heterogeneous with respect to diagnosis and IQ. In addition to anxiety, most had hyperactivity, irritability, hostility, impulsivity, and insomnia; 9 children received concurrent individual therapy and 7 received other medications, mainly anticonvulsants. Chlordiazepoxide was begun in divided doses totalling 15 mg daily and titrated individually. Maintenance dosage for periods of up to 10 months ranged from 15 to 40 mg/day (mean 26 mg). Twelve patients (23.5 percent) showed complete remission of symptoms. An additional 22 (43.1 percent) showed moderate improvement. Children with adjustment disorders in particular, improved. Of the 12 patients with mental deficiency, 3 showed marked and 3 showed moderate remissions. Side effects were relatively infrequent.

In 9 subjects diagnosed as psychoneurotic, diazepam had slight therapeutic effects. Lucas and Pasley (1969) administered this drug to 12 day care and inpatient children (8 boys, 4 girls) aged 7 to 17 years (mean 12.3 years) in a double-blind, placebo-controlled design. Ten subjects were diagnosed psychoneurotic and 2 were schizophrenic. All had moderate or high anxiety levels. Several were markedly defiant and had poor peer relationships; a few were highly aggressive. Diazepam was begun at 2.5 mg twice daily and increased until a therapeutic response or side effects occurred; 20 mg daily was the maximum dose. Diazepam and placebo conditions of varying durations occurred over the 16-week study. Three children, including the 2 schizophrenics, dropped out of the study. Subjects were rated on ten behavioral characteristics: hyperactivity, anxiety and tension, oppositional behavior, aggressiveness, impulsivity, relationship to peers and relationship to adults, need for limit setting, response to limit setting, and participation in the program. There was no significant difference between drug and placebo on any item. However, when scores on all variables were combined, subjects on diazepam improved significantly (p < 0.05) compared with subjects on placebo. On a global rating scale, 5 subjects showed no change, 2 were somewhat more anxious, and 4 were definitely worse on diazepam than placebo. Based on this study and other clinical experience, these authors felt diazepam was *not* useful in reducing anxiety or symptoms of acting out behavior in children and young adolescents, although it seemed to be useful in treating anxiety in late adolescence.

Five patients experienced somnolence, 2 had excessive salivation, 1 had tremor, 1 had dizziness, and 1 had blurred vision.

Kraft et al. (1965) concluded that chlordiazepoxide in doses of 20 to 130 mg daily was effective in decreasing anxiety and "emotional overload" in 130 behaviorally disordered children and adolescents. In 40.8 percent of the children, symptoms of hyperactivity, fears, night terrors, enuresis, reading and speech problems, truancy, and disturbed or bizarre behavior were moderately improved or eliminated, but it is noteworthy that 50 percent of those with organic brain damage worsened and 28.6 percent showed minimal or no benefit; none had an excellent response.

Bartůňková et al. (1972) compared diazepam (10 mg t.i.d.) with propericiazin (5 mg t.i.d.), chlorpromazine (25 mg t.i.d.), and placebo in a double-blind study in 21 children ages 10 to 15. Most were behaviorally disturbed boys. Target symptoms were behavioral disturbances, motor restlessness, disturbed concentration, and insubordination. The effects of diazepam did not differ significantly from placebo.

Petti et al. (1982) administered chlordiazepoxide to 9 boys; 5 had conduct disorder (3 with borderline features), 3 had personality disorder (1 with borderline features) and 1 was schizophrenic. Their ages ranged from 84 to 132 months (mean 116 months). The target symptoms were anxiety, depression, and impulsivity or explosiveness. The boys had failed to respond to three weeks of hospital milieu and placebo therapy. On optimal doses (15 to 120 mg/day, or 0.58 to 5.28 mg/kg/day) there was marked improvement in 2 boys, improvement in 4, and no change or worsening in 3 boys. The major improvements were increased verbal production, increased rapidity of thought associations and a shift from blunted affect or depressed mood to animation and a subjective sense of feeling better. Chlordiazepoxide had the most positive effect on children who were withdrawn, inhibited, anergic, depressed, and anxious. The schizophrenic child and 2 children with severe impulsivity and aggressiveness showed worsening of symptoms.

In two open studies chlordiazepoxide was reported to be effective in children with school phobia (D'Amato, 1962; Kraft et al., 1965). Klein et al. (1980) noted that children with school phobia whose separation anxiety had responded to treatment with imipramine might still refuse to go to school because they remained immobilized by anticipatory anxiety. Small doses of a benzodiazepine (for example, 5 to 10 mg of diazepam) might be useful in alleviating anticipatory anxiety in these children and assist them to venture forth on their own. Klein et al. (1980) reported adolescents with anticipatory anxiety were similarly helped.

IMMEDIATE AND LONG-TERM UNTOWARD EFFECTS

Most side effects of benzodiazepines are dose-related. The benzodiazepines are CNS depressants, particularly in higher doses, and the most common side effects are manifestations of CNS depression such as drowsiness, oversedation, fatigue, ataxia, and confusion. A grand mal seizure was reported following withdrawal in a retarded child who had not previously experienced seizures (Pilkington, 1961). Kraft et al. (1965) reported that 36 (28 percent) of their 130 patients had untoward effects. In 14 cases, side effects were slight and transient, or responded to a lowering of the dosage; in 22 cases they significantly interfered with the therapeutic efficacy of the drug. Petti et al. (1982) reported that above-optimal doses of chlordiazepoxide caused decreased animation, lethargy, or tiredness in 8 of 9 boys; 5 showed slow or slurred speech; 3 had ataxia, diplopia, or tremor; 4 developed extreme mood lability, and 3 showed increased delusions. Frommer (1967) noted that chlordiazepoxide may exacerbate depression in some cases.

"*Paradoxical reactions*" may occur, usually within the first two weeks of treatment or following a dosage increase. This may include acute excitation, increased anxiety, hallucinations, increased aggression and hostility, acute rage reactions, insomnia, and sleep disturbances (including disturbing dreams).

Three girls who received phenelzine and chlordiazepoxide had to be withdrawn from a medication trial when they developed hysterical behavior (Frommer, 1967). Thirteen (10 percent) of behaviorally disordered children ages 6 to 14 developed paradoxical reactions following administration of chlordiazepoxide; these included rage reaction, continuous crying, insomnia, and loss of all control and "going wild" (Kraft et al., 1965). In adults, sexual inappropriateness, criminal activities, or excessive uncontrolled emotional outbursts were reported (Lader, 1984). For review of the untoward effects, Greenblatt and Shader (1974), Baldessarini (1980), and Lader (1984) are recommended.

7

OTHER AGENTS

ANTISEROTONERGIC AGENTS

Because about 30 percent of autistic children, mainly those with lower IQs, have elevated serotonin levels in blood (Campbell et al., 1975; Hanley et al., 1977; Ritvo et al., 1970), attempts were made to investigate the interaction of biochemical abnormality, psychopathology, and clinical response to drug (for review, see Campbell et al., 1981). L-Dopa appeared to be promising: increases in play, energy and motor initiation, and decreases in negativism were observed (Campbell et al., 1976). However, at and above therapeutic doses, increases of preexisting stereotypies, stereotypies de novo, vomiting, worsening of irritability, motor retardation, and decrease of appetite were also seen. There was no relationship between baseline serotonin levels and clinical response in this small sample (N = 12) of subjects. More recently, administration of fenfluramine was reported to be effective in decreasing a variety of symptoms in the motor and language area, and to be associated with decreases in withdrawal and with increases in social awareness and appropriate use of language, as well as improved sleep pattern when administered over 4 months to 14 subjects (Ritvo et al., 1983). The symptoms recurred when a switch to placebo was made, and again decreased when fenfluramine therapy was reinstituted and maintained over eight months, at doses of 0.75 mg/kg twice daily (Ritvo et al., 1984). Baseline serotonin levels did not predict response to drug: decreases of symptoms were reported in subjects who had either normal or high baseline serotonin levels (Ritvo et al., 1983). However, the subgroup of respondents consisted of autistics who had low baseline serotonin levels and higher IQs (Ritvo et al., 1984). IQ tests were administered monthly throughout the studies. The reported increases in IQs appear to be a function of practice effect, and, perhaps, of maturational gains in language. Untoward effects included lethargy and decreases in appetite and weight. In an open study involving 10 hospitalized autistic children ages 3 to 5.75 years, fenfluramine, when given over a period of one to two months in doses of 1.1 to 1.8 mg/kg/day, had a mixture of tranquilizing and stimulating therapeutic effects (Campbell et al., 1986). These findings remain to be replicated in larger patient employing careful designs and assessment methods.

FOOD ADDITIVES

The claim that hyperkinesis is associated with diets containing "food additives" (e.g., artificial flavors and colors, and salicylates; Feingold, 1974) was not confirmed in subsequent studies, although this issue remains unresolved. In well-designed studies, less than about 5 percent of hyperactive children are behaviorally sensitive to food additives (Conners, 1980).

MEGAVITAMINS

High doses of vitamins are sometimes used, both in infantile autism and in attention deficit disorder with hyperactivity, though their efficacy has not been demonstrated (Arnold et al., 1978; Barness, 1976).

ANTIEPILEPTICS

There is no well-documented evidence that these drugs are effective in reducing behavioral symptoms in the absence of clinical seizure disorders (Conners & Werry, 1979; Stores, 1978).

CAFFEINE

In their review of seven controlled studies examining the effects of caffeine in hyperactive children, Klein et al. (1980) reported that only weak and inconsistently positive effects were found. They concluded that caffeine lacked sufficient therapeutic efficacy to be useful in treating hyperactive children.

8

CONCLUSIONS

A variety of drugs of different classes has been used in the treatment of disturbed children and adolescents since 1937, when the stimulant amphetamine was first introduced for the treatment of children with behavioral disorders. Our most extensive knowledge is in the area of hyperactive syndrome and stimulant medications. Over the past ten years, systematic and carefully controlled studies in autism and conduct disorder have increased our understanding of the actions of neuroleptics in these children. A conference sponsored by the National Institute of Mental Health (NIMH) in 1975 on depression in children, the proceedings of which were published in 1977 (Schulterbrandt & Raskin), gave the impetus for research into the nosology, etiology, epidemiology, and pharmacotherapy of this condition. A large number of studies, particularly in the prepubertal age group, are now rapidly contributing to our knowledge of the efficacy and safety of tricyclics in prepubertal depressives. These studies have shown that the measurement of steady-state plasma tricyclic levels can guide dosage regulation, account for treatment-nonresponders, and help to avoid the emergence of dangerous toxicity. Finally, systematic studies of lithium have begun in aggressive conduct disorder children. If this drug is shown to be effective and safe when administered on a maintenance basis, it could be a superior alternative agent to the neuroleptics because of its lack of association with tardive dyskinesia. Critical assessment of the efficacy of psychoactive drugs in schizophrenic disorders occurring in childhood and adolescence remains to be done. On the basis of a few published studies and our clinical experience, neuroleptics are less effective in attenuating target symptoms in this young age group compared to their efficacy in adult schizophrenic patients.

Despite the variety of available agents, the rationale for the pharmacotherapy of most childhood disorders is not based on the elucidation of specific biochemical abnormalities. Although all patients within a current diagnostic category share many descriptive features in common, they may be quite heterogeneous with respect to etiology. This heterogeneity with respect to etiology could account for some of the individual differences in response to the same medication. The existence of mutually exclusive subgroups of responders to one particular type of medication and not to another could provide valuable clues to specific underlying biochemical abnormalities.

In adult psychiatric patients, the advent of psychopharmacology and subsequent collaborative studies sponsored by the Psychopharmacology Research Branch of the NIMH required diagnostically homogeneous patient samples. This forced a critical appraisal of existing diagnostic categories and further refinement of diagnostic criteria, in order to promote communication between researchers (Feighner et al., 1972; Spitzer et al., 1978). Further advancements in childhood psychopharmacology will depend upon continuous refinements of diagnostic nosology and, perhaps, identification of biochemical abnormalities in specific disorders. In addition, in some conditions, the more widespread availability of drug levels in blood may ensure that patients are treated with adequate dosages of medication.

In view of the complexity of most childhood disorders, it is not surprising that interventions based on a single modality rarely produce dramatic therapeutic results. Therefore, additional studies should be designed to assess critically and to compare pharmacotherapy and psychosocial interventions, including behavior and psychotherapy, and evaluate their possible interactions. To date, only a few examples of this type of approach exist; these studies involved samples of hyperactive (Gittelman-Klein, Klein, Abikoff et al., 1976), autistic (Campbell, Anderson et al., 1978) and enuretic children (McConaghy, 1969). It is hoped that comprehensive treatment programs consisting of multiple and complementary interventions, which have demonstrated efficacy and superiority over individual methods of treatment, will result. Another neglected area that may be useful to consider in future research is the development of interventions to enhance cognitive performance. Effective interventions of this type may be of special benefit to mentally retarded children and children with developmental disorders.

Future areas of research should consider reasons for the seemingly lesser effectiveness of neuroleptics in the treatment of schizophrenic disorder occurring in childhood and early adolescence compared with the condition in adults. Perhaps this issue will be elucidated as research continues in the development of alternative interventions that are not focused on dopaminergic blockade. Furthermore, if an alternative and effective nondopaminergic intervention were to be found, this might contribute to a resolution of the problem of tardive dyskinesia occurring with chronic neuroleptic administration. The recognition and existence of tardive dyskinesia in children should serve as an important reminder to investigators in this field. The introduction of effective measures to prevent or treat the emergence of tardive dyskinesia has become one of the greatest challenges for future investigators. For the present, we must remain vigilant for the possible emergence of late and undesirable features of our interventions.

REFERENCES

Achenbach, T. M. (1978). Psychopathology of childhood: Research problems and issues. *Journal of Consulting and Clinical Psychology, 46,* 759-776.

Achenbach, T. M., & Edelbrock, C. S. (1979). The child behavior profile: II. Boys aged 12-16 and girls aged 6-11 and 12-16. *Journal of Consulting and Clinical Psychology, 47,* 223-233.

Alexandris, A., & Lundell, F. W. (1968). Effect of thioridazine, amphetamine, and placebo on the hyperkinetic syndrome and cognitive area in mentally deficient children. *Canadian Medical Association Journal, 98,* 92-96.

Aman, M. G. (1978). Drugs, learning and the psychotherapies. In J. S. Werry (Ed.), *Pediatric psychopharmacology: The use of behavior modifying drugs in children.* New York: Brunner/Mazel.

Aman, M. G. (1984). Drugs and learning in mentally retarded persons. In G. D. Burrows & J. S. Werry (Eds.), *Advances in human psychopharmacology* (Vol. 3). Greenwich, CT: JAI Press.

Aman, M. G., & Werry, J. S. (1982). Methylphenidate and diazepam in severe reading retardation. *Journal of the American Academy of Child Psychiatry, 21*(1), 31-37.

American Psychiatric Association Mental Hospital Service. (1952). *Diagnostic and statistical manual (DSM). Mental disorders.* Washington, DC: Author.

American Psychiatric Association. (1968). *Diagnostic and statistical manual of mental disorders* (2nd ed.) (DSM-II). Washington, DC: Author.

American Psychiatric Association. (1980). *Diagnostic and statistical manual of mental disorders* (3rd ed.). (DSM-III). Washington, DC: Author.

Anderson, L. T., Campbell, M., Grega, D. M., Perry, R., Small, A. M., & Green, W. H. (1984). Haloperidol in the treatment of infantile autism: Effects on learning and behavioral symptoms. *American Journal of Psychiatry, 141*(10), 1195-1202.

Annell, A.-L. (1969a). Lithium in the treatment of children and adolescents. *Acta Psychiatrica Scandinavica, 207,* (supplement) 19-30.

Annell, A.-L. (1969b). Manic-depressive illness in children and effect of treatment with lithium carbonate. *Acta Paedopsychiatrica, 36,* 292-301.

Arnold, L. E., Christopher, J., Huestis, R. D., & Smeltzer, D. J. (1978). Megavitamins for minimal brain dysfunction: A placebo controlled study. *Journal of the American Medical Association, 240,* 2642-2643.

Baldessarini, R. J. (1980). Drugs and the treatment of psychiatric disorders. In A. G. Gilman, L. S. Goodman, & A. Gilman (Eds.), *The pharmacological basis of therapeutics* (6th ed.). New York: Macmillan.

Baldessarini, R. J., & Stephens, J. H. (1970). Clinical pharmacology and toxicology of lithium salts. *Archives of General Psychiatry, 22,* 72-77.

Ballinger, C. T., Varley, C. K., & Nolen, P. A. (1984). Effects of methylphenidate on reading in children with attention deficit disorder. *American Journal of Psychiatry, 141,* 1590-1593.

Barness, L. A. (1976). Megavitamin therapy for childhood psychoses and learning disabilities. *Pediatrics, 58,* 910-911.

Bartůňková, Z., Černý, L., Ortilová, J., & Šturma, J. (1972). Propericiazin, diazepam, chlorpromazine and placebo in a double-blind trial in pedopsychiatric therapy. *Activitas Nervosa Superior* (Praha) *14*(2), 83-84.

Belfer, M. L., & Shader, R. I. (1970). Autonomic effects. In R. I. Shader & A. DiMascio (Eds.), *Psychotropic drug side effects.* Baltimore: Williams & Wilkins Company.

Bennett, W. G., Korein, J., Kalmijn, M., Grega, D. M., & Campbell, M. (1983). EEG and treatment of hospitalized aggressive children with haloperidol or lithium. *Biological Psychiatry, 18*(12), 1427-1440.

Berg, I., Hullin, R., Allsopp, M., O'Brien, P., & MacDonald, R. (1974). Bipolar manic-depressive psychosis in early adolescence: A case report. *British Journal of Psychiatry, 125,* 416-417.

Berger, P. A., & Rexroth, K. (1980). Tardive dyskinesia: Clinical, biological, and pharmacological perspectives. *Schizophrenia Bulletin, 6*(1), 102-116.

Bigger, J. T., Jr., Kantor, S. J., Glassman, A. H., & Perel, J. M. (1978). Cardiovascular effects of tricyclic antidepressant drugs. In M. A. Lipton, A. DiMascio, & K. F. Killam (Eds.), *Psychopharmacology: A generation of progress.* New York: Raven Press.

Blackwell, B. (1982). Treatment compliance. In J. H. Greist, J. W. Jefferson, & R. L. Spitzer (Eds.), *Treatment of mental disorders.* New York: Oxford University Press.

Bogomolny, A., Erenberg, G., & Rothner, A. D. (1982). Behavioral effects of haloperidol in young Tourette syndrome patients. In A. J. Friedhoff and T. N. Chase (Eds.), *Advances in neurology, (Vol. 35), Gilles de la Tourette Syndrome.* New York: Raven Press.

Bradford Hill, A. (1971). *Principles of medical statistics.* New York: Oxford University Press.

Bradley, C. (1937). The behavior of children receiving benzedrine. *American Journal of Psychiatry, 94,* 577-585.

Bradley, C., & Bowen, M. (1940). School performance of children receiving amphetamine (benzedrine) sulfate. *American Journal of Orthopsychiatry, 10,* 782-788.

Breitner, C. (1962). An approach to the treatment of juvenile delinquency. *Arizona Medicine, 19,* 82-87.

Brown, D., Winsberg, B., Bialer, I., & Press, M. (1973). Imipramine therapy and seizures. *American Journal of Psychiatry, 130,* 210-212.

Brumback, R. A., & Weinberg, W. A. (1977). Mania in childhood. *American Journal of Diseases of Childhood, 131,* 1122-1126.

Burdock, E. I. (1982). Problems and profits of quantitative evaluation. In E. I. Burdock, A. Sudilovsky, & S. Gershon (Eds.), *The behavior of psychiatric patients.* New York: Marcel Dekker.

Burdock, E. I., & Hardesty, A. S. (1967). Contrasting behavior patterns of mentally retarded and emotionally disturbed children. In J. Zubin & J. A. Jervis (Eds.), *Psychopathology of mental development.* New York: Grune & Stratton.

Buss, A. H., & Durkee, A. (1957). An inventory for assessing different kinds of hostility. *Journal of Consulting Psychology, 21*(8), 343-349.

Campbell, M. (1979). Psychopharmacology for children and adolescents. In J. D. Noshpitz (Ed.), *Basic handbook of child psychiatry (Vol. 3).* New York: Basic Books.

Campbell, M. (1985). Pervasive developmental disorders: Autistic and schizophrenic disorders. In J. M. Wiener (Ed.), *Psychopharmacology of childhood and adolescence.* New York: John Wiley.

Campbell, M., Anderson, L. T., Cohen, I. L., Perry, R., Small, A. M., Green, W. H., Anderson, L., & McCandless, W. (1982). Haloperidol in autistic children: Effects on learning, behavior and abnormal involuntary movements. *Psychopharmacology Bulletin, 18*(1), 110-112.

Campbell, M., Anderson, L. T., Deutsch, S. I., & Green, W. H. (1984). Psychopharmacological treatment of children with the syndrome of autism. *Pediatric Annals, 13,* 309-316.

Campbell, M., Anderson, L. T., Meier, M., Cohen, I. L., Small, A. M., Samit, C., & Sachar, E. J. (1978). A comparison of haloperidol, behavior therapy and their interaction in autistic children. *Journal of the American Academy of Child Psychiatry, 17*(4), 640-655.

Campbell, M., Anderson, L. T., Small, A. M., Perry, R., Green, W. H., & Caplan, R. (1982). The effects of haloperidol on learning and behavior in autistic children. *Journal of Autism and Developmental Disorders, 12*(2), 167-175.

Campbell, M., Cohen, I. L., & Anderson, L. T. (1981). Pharmacotherapy for autistic children: A summary of research. *Canadian Journal of Psychiatry, 26,* 265-273.

Campbell, M., Cohen, I. L., & Small, A. M. (1982). Drugs in aggressive behavior. *Journal of the American Academy of Child Psychiatry, 21,* 107-117.

Campbell, M., Deutsch, S. I., Perry, R., Wolsky, B., Palij, M., & Lukashok, D. (1986). Short-term efficacy and safety of fenfluramine in hospitalized preschool-age autistic children: an open study. *Psychopharmacology Bulletin, 22*(1).

Campbell, M., Fish, B., David, R., Shapiro, T., Collins, P., & Koh, C. (1972). Response to triiodothyronine and dextroamphetamine: A study of preschool schizophrenic children. *Journal of Autism and Childhood Schizophrenia, 2*(4), 343-358.

Campbell, M., Fish, B., Korein, J., Shapiro, T., Collins, P., & Koh, C. (1972). Lithium and chlorpromazine: A controlled crossover study of hyperactive severely disturbed young children. *Journal of Autism and Childhood Schizophrenia, 2*(3), 234-263.

Campbell, M., Fish, B., Shapiro, T., & Floyd, A., Jr. (1970). Thiothixene in young disturbed children: A pilot study. *Archives of General Psychiatry, 23,* 70-72.

Campbell, M., Fish, B., Shapiro, T., & Floyd, A., Jr. (1971). Study of molindone in disturbed preschool children. *Current Therapeutic Research, 13,* 28-33.

Campbell, M., Fish, B., Shapiro, T., & Floyd, A., Jr. (1972). Acute responses of schizophrenic children to a sedative and a "stimulating" neuroleptic: A pharmacologic yardstick. *Current Therapeutic Research, 14*(12), 759-766.

Campbell, M., Friedman, E., Green, W. H., Collins, P. J., Small, A. M., & Breuer, H. (1975). Blood serotonin in schizophrenic children. A preliminary study. *International Pharmacopsychiatry, 10,* 213-221.

Campbell, M., Green, W. H., Caplan, R., & David, R. (1982). Psychiatry and endocrinology in children. Early infantile autism and psychosocial dwarfism. In P.J.V. Beaumont & G. D. Burrows (Eds.), *Handbook of psychiatry and endocrinology.* Amsterdam: Elsevier Biomedical Press.

Campbell, M., Green, W. H., Perry, R., & Anderson, L. T. (1983). Pharmacotherapy. In C. E. Walker & M. C. Roberts (Eds.), *Handbook of clinical child psychology.* New York: John Wiley.

Campbell, M., Grega, D. M., Green, W. H., & Bennett, W. G. (1983). Neuroleptic-induced dyskinesias in children. *Clinical Neuropharmacology, 6,* 207-222.

Campbell, M., Perry, R., Bennett, W. G., Small, A. M., Green, W. H., Grega, D., Schwartz, V., & Anderson, L. (1983). Long-term therapeutic efficacy and drug-related abnormal movements: A prospective study of haloperidol in autistic children. *Psychopharmacology Bulletin, 19*(1), 80-83.

Campbell, M., Perry, R., & Green, W. H. (1984). Use of lithium in children and adolescents. *Psychosomatics, 25*(2), 95-106.

Campbell, M., Petti, T. A., Green, W. H., Cohen, I. L., Genieser, N. B., & David, R. (1980). Some physical parameters of young autistic children. *Journal of the American Academy of Child Psychiatry, 19,* 193-212.

Campbell, M., Small, A. M., Collins, P. J., Friedman, E., David, R., & Genieser, N. (1976). Levodopa and levoamphetamine: A crossover study in young schizophrenic children. *Current Therapeutic Research, 19*(1), 70-86.

Campbell, M., Small, A. M., Green, W. H., Jennings, S. J., Perry, R., Bennett, W. G., & Anderson, L. (1984). Behavioral efficacy of haloperidol and lithium carbonate: A comparison in hospitalized aggressive children with conduct disorder. *Archives of General Psychiatry, 41*(7), 650-656.

Campbell, M., Small, A. M., Hollander, C. S., Korein, J., Cohen, I. L., Kalmijn, M., & Ferris, S. (1978). A controlled crossover study of triiodothyronine in autistic children. *Journal of Autism and Childhood Schizophrenia, 8,* 371-381.

Carlson, G. A., & Cantwell, D. P. (1979). A survey of depressive symptoms in a child and adolescent psychiatric population. *Journal of the American Academy of Child Psychiatry, 18,* 587-599.

Carlson, G. A., & Strober, M. (1978). Manic-depressive illness in early adolescence. *Journal of the American Academy of Child Psychiatry, 17,* 138-153.

Carroll, B. J. (1978). Neuroendocrine function in psychiatric disorders. In M. A. Lipton, A. DiMascio, & K. F. Killam (Eds.), *Psychopharmacology: A generation of progress.* New York: Raven Press.

Chambers, W., Puig-Antich, J., & Tabrizi, M. A. (1978). *The ongoing development of the Kiddie-SADS (Schedule for affective disorders and schizophrenia for school-age children).* Paper presented at the Annual Meeting of the American Academy of Child Psychiatry, San Francisco.

Charney, D. S., Menkes, D. B., & Heninger, G. R. (1981). Receptor sensitivity and the mechanism of action of antidepressant treatment: Implications for the etiology and therapy of depression. *Archives of General Psychiatry, 38,* 1160-1180.

Chassan, J. B. (1979). *Research design in clinical psychology and psychiatry* (2nd ed.). New York: Irvington Publishers.

Chien, C.-P., Jung, K., & Ross-Townsend, A. (1980). Methodological approach to the measurement of tardive dyskinesia: Piezoelectric recording and concurrent validity test of five clinical rating scales. In W. E. Fann, R. C. Smith, J. M. Davies, & E. F. Domino (Eds.), *Tardive dyskinesia. Research & Treatment.* New York: SP Medical & Scientific Books.

Chouinard, G., & Jones, B. D. (1980). Neuroleptic-induced supersensitivity psychosis: Clinical and pharmacological characteristics. *American Journal of Psychiatry, 137,* 16-21.

Cochran, W. G., & Cox, G. M. (1957). *Experimental designs* (2nd ed.). New York: John Wiley.

Coffey, B., Shader, R. I., & Greenblatt, D. J. (1983). Pharmacokinetics of benzodiazepines and psychostimulants in children. *Journal of Clinical Psychopharmacology, 3*(4), 217-225.

Cohen, I. L., Campbell, M., Posner, D., Small, A. M., Triebel, D., & Anderson, L. T. (1980). Behavioral effects of haloperidol in young autistic children: An objective analysis using a within-subjects reversal design. *Journal of the American Academy of Child Psychiatry, 19,* 665-677.

Cohen, W. J., & Cohen, N. H. (1974). Lithium carbonate, haloperidol, and irreversible brain damage. *Journal of the American Medical Association, 230,* 1283-1287.

Comings, D. E., & Comings, B. G. (1984). Tourette's syndrome and attention deficit with hyperactivity: Are they genetically related? *Journal of the American Academy of Child Psychiatry, 23,* 138-146.

Conners, C. K. (1969). A teacher rating scale for use in drug studies with children. *American Journal of Psychiatry, 126,* 152-156.

Conners, C. K. (1980). *Food additives and hyperactive children.* New York: Plenum Press.

Conners, C. K. (1985). Methodological and Assessment Issues in Pediatric Psychopharmacology. In J. M. Weiner (Ed.), *Psychopharmacology in Childhood and Adolescence.* New York: John Wiley.

Conners, C. K., Eisenberg, L., & Barcai, A. (1967). Effect of dextroamphetamine on children. Studies on subjects with learning disabilities and school behavior problems. *Archives of General Psychiatry, 17,* 478-485.

Conners, C. K., Rothschild, G., Eisenberg, L., Schwartz, L. S., & Robinson, E. (1969). Dextroamphetamine sulfate in children with learning disorders. Effects on perception, learning, and achievement. *Archives of General Psychiatry, 21,* 182-190.

Conners, C. K., & Taylor, E. (1980). Pemoline, methylphenidate, and placebo in children with minimal brain dysfunction. *Archives of General Psychiatry, 37,* 922-930.

Conners, C. K., Taylor, E., Meo, G., Kurtz, M. A., & Fournier, M. (1972). Magnesium pemoline and dextroamphetamine: A controlled study in children with minimal brain dysfunction. *Psychopharmacologia, 26,* 321-336.

Conners, C. K., & Werry, J. S. (1979). Pharmacotherapy. In H. C. Quay & J. S. Werry (Eds.), *Psychopathological disorders of childhood* (2nd ed.). New York: John Wiley.

Crane, G. E., & Naranjo, E. R. (1971). Motor disorders induced by neuroleptics. *Archives of General Psychiatry, 24*(2), 179-184.

Crane, G. E., & Smeets, R. A. (1974). Tardive dyskinesia and drug therapy in geriatric patients. *Archives of General Psychiatry, 30*(3), 341-343.

Cunningham, M. A., Pillai, V., Rogers, W.J.B. (1968). Haloperidol in the treatment of children with severe behaviour disorders. *British Journal of Psychiatry, 114,* 845-854.

Dale, P. G. (1980). Lithium therapy in aggressive mentally subnormal patients. *British Journal of Psychiatry, 137,* 469-474.

D'Amato, G. (1962). Chlordiazepoxide in management of school phobia. *Diseases of the Nervous System, 23,* 292-295.

Davis, J. M. (1985). Antipsychotic drugs. In H. I. Kaplan & B. J. Sadock (Eds.), *Comprehensive textbook of psychiatry/IV.* Baltimore: Williams & Wilkins.

Debray, P., Messerschmitt, P., Lonchap, D., & Herbault, M. (1972). L'utilization du pimozide en pédopsychiatrie. *Nouvelle Presse Medicale, 1* (part 3), 2917-2918.

DeLong, G. R. (1978). Lithium carbonate treatment of select behavior disorders in children suggesting manic-depressive illness. *The Journal of Pediatrics, 93*(4), 689-694.

DeLong, G. R., & Nieman, G. W. (1983). Lithium-induced behavior changes in children with symptoms suggesting manic-depressive illness. *Psychopharmacology Bulletin, 19*(2), 258-265.

Denckla, M. B., Bemporad, J. R., & MacKay, M. C. (1976). Tics following methylphenidate administration: A report of 20 cases. *Journal of the American Medical Association, 235*(13), 1349-1351.

Deutsch, S. I., & Campbell, M. (1984). *The relationship of biochemical abnormalities and clinical response to type of neuroleptic in infantile autism.* Paper presented at the 31st Annual Meeting of the American Academy of Child Psychiatry, Toronto.

Die Trill, M. L., Wolsky, B. B., Shell, J., Green, W. H., Perry, R., & Campbell, M. (1984). *Effects of long term haloperidol treatment on intellectual functioning in autistic children: A pilot study.* Paper presented at the 31st Annual Meeting of the American Academy of Child Psychiatry, Toronto.

DiMascio, A., & Shader, R. I. (1970). Behavioral toxicity. Part I: Definition. Part II: Psychomotor functions. In R. I. Shader & A. DiMascio (Eds.), *Psychotropic drug side effects*. Baltimore: Williams & Wilkins.

DiMascio, A., Shader, R. I., & Giller, D. R. (1970). Behavioral toxicity. Part III: Perceptual-cognitive functions. Part IV: Emotional (mood) states. In R. I. Shader & A. DiMascio (Eds.), *Psychotropic drug side effects*. Baltimore: Williams & Wilkins.

DiMascio, A., Shader, R. I., & Harmatz, J. S. (1970). Behavioral toxicity. Part V: Gross behavior patterns. In R. I. Shader & A. DiMascio (Eds.), *Psychotropic drug side effects*. Baltimore: Williams & Wilkins.

Dostal, T. (1972). Antiaggressive effect of lithium salts in mentally retarded adolescents. In A.-L. Annell (Ed.), *Depressive states in childhood and adolescence*. Stockholm: Almqvist & Wiksell.

Dyson, W. L., & Barcai, A. (1970). Treatment of children of lithium-responding parents. *Current Therapeutic Research, 12*(5), 286-290.

Ebert, M. H., & Shader, R. I. (1970a). Cardiovascular effects. In R. I. Shader & A. DiMascio (Eds.), *Psychotropic drug side effects*. Baltimore: Williams & Wilkins.

Ebert, M. H., & Shader, R. I. (1970b). Hematological effects. In R. I. Shader & A. DiMascio (Eds.), *Psychotropic drug side effects*. Baltimore: Williams & Wilkins.

Ebert, M. H., & Shader, R. I. (1970c). Hepatic effects. In R. I. Shader & A. DiMascio (Eds.), *Psychotropic drug side effects*. Baltimore: Williams & Wilkins.

Ederer, F. (Ed.). (1975). The randomized controlled clinical trial. *American Journal of Opthalmology, 79*(5), 752-789.

Eggins, L., Barker, P., & Walker, R. J. (1975). A study of the heights and weights of different groups of disturbed children. *Child Psychiatry and Human Development, 5*(4), 203-208.

Engelhardt, D. M., & Polizos, P. (1978). Adverse effects of pharmacotherapy in childhood psychosis. In M. A. Lipton, A. DiMascio, & K. F. Killam (Eds.), *Psychopharmacology: A Generation of Progress*. New York: Raven Press.

Engelhardt, D. M., Polizos, P., Waizer, J., & Hoffman, S. P. (1973). A double-blind comparison of fluphenazine and haloperidol. *Journal of Autism and Childhood Schizophrenia, 3*, 128-137.

Engelsmann, F. (1982). Design of psychometric instruments: item construction, scaling, reliability and validity, norms. In E. I. Burdock, A. Sudilovsky, & S. Gershon (Eds.), *The Behavior of Psychiatric Patients*. New York: Marcel Dekker.

Fann, W. E., Smith, R. C., Davis, J. M., & Domino, E. F. (Eds.). (1980). *Tardive Dyskinesia. Research & Treatment*. Jamaica, New York: Spectrum.

Fann, W. E., Stafford, J. R., Malone, R. L., Frost, J. D., & Richman, B. W. (1977). Clinical research techniques in tardive dyskinesia. *American Journal of Psychiatry, 134*(7), 759-762.

Faretra, G., Dooher, L., & Dowling, J. (1970). Comparison of haloperidol and fluphenazine in disturbed children. *American Journal of Psychiatry, 126*, 1670-1673.

Feighner, J. P., Robins, E., Guze, S. B., Woodruff, R. A., Winokur, G., & Munoz, R. (1972). Diagnostic criteria for use in psychiatric research. *Archives of General Psychiatry, 26*, 57-63.

Feingold, B. F. (1974). *Hyperkinesis and learning difficulties (H-LD) linked to the ingestion of artifical colors and flavors*. Paper presented at the annual meeting of the American Medical Association, section on allergy, Chicago.

Feinstein, S. C., & Wolpert, E. A. (1973). Juvenile manic-depressive illness. *Journal of the American Academy of Child Psychiatry, 12*, 123-136.

Fink, M. (1978). Psychoactive drugs and the waking EEG, 1966-1976. In M. A. Lipton, A. DiMascio, & K. F. Killam (Eds.), *Psychopharmacology: A Generation of Progress.* New York: Raven Press.

Fish, B. (1968). Drug use in psychiatric disorders in children: *American Journal of Psychiatry, 124,* 31-36.

Fish, B., Campbell, M., Shapiro, T., & Weinstein, J. (1969). Preliminary findings on thiothixene compared to other drugs in psychotic children under five years. In H. E. Lehmann & T. A. Ban (Eds.), *The thioxanthenes: Modern problems of pharmacopsychiatry* (Vol. 2). Basel: S. Karger.

Fish, B., Shapiro, T., & Campbell, M. (1966). Long-term prognosis and the response of schizophrenic children to drug therapy: A controlled study of trifluoperazine. *American Journal of Psychiatry, 123,* 32-39.

Forsythe, W. I., & Redmond, A. (1970). Enuresis and the electric alarm: Study of 200 cases. *British Medical Journal, 1,* 211-213.

Forsythe, W. I., & Redmond, A. (1974). Enuresis and spontaneous cure rate. *Archives of Disease in Childhood, 49,* 259-263.

Friedhoff, A. J., & Chase, T. N. (Eds.). (1982). *Advances in Neurology, Volume 35. Gilles de la Tourette Syndrome.* New York: Raven Press.

Frommer, E. A. (1967). Treatment of childhood depression with antidepressant drugs. *British Medical Journal, 1,* 729-732.

Frommer, E. A. (1968). Depressive illness in childhood. In A. Coppen & A. Walk (Eds.), Recent developments in affective disorders: A symposium. *British Journal of Psychiatry,* Special Publication No. 2. Ashford, Kent: Headley Brothers.

Gallant, D. M., Edwards, C. G., Bishop, M. P., & Gailbraith, G. C. (1964). Withdrawal symptoms after abrupt cessation of antipsychotic compounds: Clinical confirmation in chronic schizophrenics. *American Journal of Psychiatry, 121,* 491-493.

Ganong, W. F., & Martini, L. (Eds.). (1973). *Frontiers in neuroendocrinology.* New York: Oxford University Press.

Gardos, G., & Cole, J. O. (1980a). Problems in assessment of tardive dyskinesia. In W. E. Fann, R. C. Smith, J. M. Davis, & E. F. Domino (Eds.), *Tardive dyskinesia. Research & treatment.* New York: SP Medical & Scientific Books.

Gardos, G., & Cole, J. O. (1980b). Overview: Public health issues in tardive dyskinesia. *American Journal of Psychiatry, 137*(7), 776-781.

Gardos, G., Cole, J. O., & Tarsy, D. (1978). Withdrawal syndromes associated with antipsychotic drugs. *American Journal of Psychiatry, 135*(11), 1321-1324.

Gardos, G., Cole, J. O., & La Brie, R. (1977). The assessment of tardive dyskinesia. *Archives of General Psychiatry, 34,* 1206-1212.

Gardos, G., DiMascio, A., Salzman, C., & Shader, R. I. (1968). Differential actions of chlordiazepoxide and oxazepam on hostility. *Archives of General Psychiatry, 18,* 757-760.

Garfield, S. L. (1982). Psychological assessment. In E. I. Burdock, A. Sudilovsky, & S. Gershon (Eds.), *The behavior of psychiatric patients.* New York: Marcel Dekker.

Geller, B., Guttmacher, L. B., & Bleeg, M. (1981). Coexistence of childhood onset pervasive developmental disorder and attention deficit disorder with hyperactivity. *American Journal of Psychiatry, 13,* 388-389.

Geller, B., Perel, J. M., Knitter, E. F., Lycaki, H., & Farooki, Z. Q. (1983). Nortriptyline in major depressive disorder in children: Response, steady-state plasma levels, predictive kinetics, and pharmacokinetics. *Psychopharmacology Bulletin, 19,* 62-65.

General Considerations for the Clinical Evaluation of Drugs. (1977). FDA 77-3040, Department of Health, Education and Welfare, Public Health Service, Food and Drug Administration (1977). Washington, DC: Government Printing Office.

Gerlach, J., & Faurbye, A. (1980). Pathophysiological aspects of reversible and irreversible tardive dyskinesia. In W. E. Fann, R. C. Smith, J. M. Davis, & E. F. Domino (Eds.), *Tardive dyskinesia. Research & treatment.* New York: Spectrum Publications.

Gershon, S. (1973). Clinical standards in pediatric psychopharmacology. *Psychopharmacology Bulletin, Special Issue, Pharmacotherapy of Children.*

Gershon, S., & Shopsin, B. (1973). *Lithium: Its role in psychiatric research and treatment.* New York: Plenum Press.

Gesell, A., & Amatruda, C. S. (1947). *Developmental diagnosis* (2nd ed.). New York: Harper & Row.

Gittelman-Klein, R. (1978). Psychopharmacological treatment of anxiety disorders, mood disorders, and Tourette's disorder in children. In M. A. Lipton, A. DiMascio, & K. F. Killam (Eds.), *Psychopharmacology: A generation of progress.* New York: Raven Press.

Gittelman-Klein, R., & Klein, D. F. (1973a). School phobia: Diagnostic considerations in the light of imipramine effects. *Journal of Nervous and Mental Disease, 156,* 199-215.

Gittelman-Klein, R., & Klein, D. F. (1973b). *The relationship between behavioral and psychological test changes in hyperkinetic children.* Presented at the 12th Annual Meeting of the American College of Neuropsychopharmacology, Palm Springs.

Gittelman-Klein, R., & Klein, D. F. (1976). Methylphenidate effects in learning disabilites. Psychometric changes. *Archives of General Psychiatry, 33,* 655-664.

Gittelman-Klein, R., Klein, D. F., Abikoff, H., Katz, S., Gloisten, A. C., & Kates, W. (1976). Relative efficacy of methylphenidate and behavior modification in hyperkinetic children: An interim report. *Journal of Abnormal Child Psychology, 4,* 361-379.

Gittelman-Klein, R., Klein, D. F., Katz, S., Saraf, K. R., & Pollack, E. (1976). Comparative effects of methylphenidate and thioridazine in hyperkinetic children: I. Clinical results. *Archives of General Psychiatry, 33,* 1217-1231.

Gittelman-Klein, R., Spitzer, R., & Cantwell, D. P. (1978). Diagnostic classifications and psychopharmacological indications. In J. S. Werry (Ed.), *Pediatric psychopharmacology. The use of behavior modifying drugs in children.* New York: Brunner/Mazel.

Glen, A.I.M., Johnson, A. L., & Shepherd, M. (1984). Continuation therapy with lithium and amitriptyline in unipolar depressive illness: A randomized, double-blind, controlled study. *Psychological Medicine, 14,* 37-50.

Gleser, G. C. (1968). Psychometric contributions to the assessment of patients. In D. H. Efron, J. O. Cole, J. Levine, & J. R. Wittenborn (Eds.), *Psychopharmacology, A review of progress, 1956-1967.* Washington, DC: Government Printing Office, Public Health Service Publication 1836.

Gleser, G. C., Gottschalk, L. A., Fox, R., & Lippert, W. (1965). Immediate changes in affect with chlordiazepoxide. *Archives of General Psychiatry, 13,* 291-295.

Glick, B. S., Schulman, D., & Turecki, S. (1971). Diazepam, (Valium) treatment in childhood sleep disorders. *Diseases of the Nervous System, 32,* 565-566.

Goetzl, U., Grunberg, F., & Berkowitz, B. (1977). Lithium carbonate in the management of hyperactive aggressive behavior of the mentally retarded. *Comprehensive Psychiatry, 18*(6), 599-606.

Gottschalk, L. A., Gleser, G. C., & Springer, K. J. (1963). Three hostility scales applicable to verbal samples. *Archives of General Psychiatry, 9*(9), 254-279.

Gough, H. (1969). *The California psychological inventory manual.* Palo Alto, CA: Consulting Psychologists Press.

Gram, L. F., & Rafaelsen, O. J. (1972). Lithium treatment of psychotic children: A controlled clinical trial. In A.-L. Annell (Ed.), *Depressive states in childhood and adolescense.* Stockholm: Almqvist & Wiksell.

Granacher, R. P. (1981). Differential diagnosis of tardive dyskinesia: An overview. *American Journal of Psychiatry, 138*(10), 1288-1297.

Green, W. H. (in press). Psychosocial dwarfism. In B. B. Lahey & A. E. Kazdin (Eds.), *Advances in clinical child psychology* (Vol. 9). New York: Plenum Press.

Green, W. H., Campbell, M., & David, R. (1984). Psychosocial dwarfism: A critical review of the evidence. *Journal of the American Academy of Child Psychiatry, 23* (1), 39-48.

Green, W. H., Campbell, M., Hardesty, A. S., Grega, D. M., Padron-Gayol, M., Shell, J., & Erlenmeyer-Kimling, L. (1984). A comparison of schizophrenic and autistic children. *Journal of the American Academy of Child Psychiatry, 23*(4), 399-409.

Green, W. H., Campbell, M., Wolsky, B. B., Deutsch, S. I., Golden, R. R., & Cicero, S. D. (1984). *Effects of short and long term haloperidol administration on growth in young autistic children.* Paper presented at the 31st Annual Meeting of the American Academy of Child Psychiatry, Toronto.

Green, W. H., Deutsch, S. I., & Campbell, M. (in press). Psychosocial dwarfism, infantile autism, and attention deficit disorder. In C. B. Nemeroff & P. T. Loosen (Eds.), *Handbook of Clinical Psychoneuroendocrinology.* New York: Guilford Press.

Greenberg, L. M., & Roth, S. (1966). Differential effects of abrupt versus gradual withdrawal of chlorpromazine in hospitalized chronic schizophrenic patients. *American Journal of Psychiatry, 123*(8), 221-226.

Greenblatt, D. J., & Shader, R. I. (1974). *Benzodiazepines in clinical practice.* New York: Raven Press.

Greenhill, L. L., Barmack, J. E., Spalten, D., Anderson, M., & Halpern, F. (1981). Molindone hydrochloride in the treatment of aggressive, hospitalized children. *Psychopharmacology Bulletin, 17*(1), 125.

Greenhill, L. L., Puig-Antich, J., Halpern, F., Sachar, E. J., Rubinstein, B., Chambers, W., Fiscina, B., & Florea, J. (1980). Growth disturbances in hyperkinetic children. [Letter to editor]. *Pediatrics, 66*(1), 152-153.

Greenhill, L. L., Rieder, R. O., Wender, P. H., Bushsbaum, M., & Zahn, T. P. (1973). Lithium carbonate in the treatment of hyperactive children. *Archives of General Psychiatry, 28,* 636-640.

Gualtieri, C. T., Barnhill, J., McGimsey, J., & Schell, D. (1980). Tardive dyskinesia and other movement disorders in children treated with psychotropic drugs. *Journal of the American Academy of Child Psychiatry, 19*(3), 491-510.

Gualtieri, C. T., Breuning, S. E., Schroeder, S. R., & Quade, D. (1982). Tardive dyskinesia in mentally retarded children, adolescents, and young adults: North Carolina and Michigan studies. *Psychopharmacology Bulletin, 18*(1), 62-65.

Gualtieri, C. T., Golden, R., Evans, R. W., & Hicks, R. E. (1984). Blood level measurement of psychoactive drugs in pediatric psychiatry. *Therapeutic Drug Monitoring, 6,* 127-141.

Gualtieri, C. T., Quade, D., Hicks, R. E., Mayo, J. P., & Schroeder, S. R. (1984). Tardive dyskinesia and other clinical consequences of neuroleptic treatment in children and adolescents. *American Journal of Psychiatry, 141*(1), 20-23.

Gualtieri, C. T., Wafgin, W., Kanoy, R., Patrick, K., Shen, D., Youngblood, W., Mueller, R., & Breese, G. (1982). Clinical studies of methylphenidate serum levels in children and adults. *Journal of the American Academy of Child Psychiatry, 21,* 19-26.

Guidelines for the Clinical Evaluation of Psychoactive Drugs in Infants and Children. (1979, July). Stock no. 017-012-00281-1, U.S. Department of Health, Education, and Welfare, Public Health Service, Food and Drug Administration. Washington, DC: Government Printing Office.

Guy, W. (1976). *ECDEU assessment manual for psychopharmacology* [rev. ed.]. Publication (ADM) 76-338. Rockville, MD: Department of Health, Education and Welfare.

Guy, W. (1982). Classification of behavioral instruments appropriate for measurement of psychopathology. In E. I. Burdock, A. Sudilovsky, & S. Gershon (Eds.), *The behavior of psychiatric patients.* New York: Marcel Dekker.

Hamill, P.V.V., Drizd, T. A., Johnson, C. L., Reed, R. B., & Roche, A. F. (1976). *N.C.H.S. Growth Charts, 1976.* Monthly Vital Statistics Report, Health Examination Survey Data. Publication (HRA) 76-1120, *25*(Suppl. 3), 1-22. Washington, DC: National Center for Health Statistics.

Hamilton, M. (1982). Types of assessment. In E. I. Burdock, A. Sudilovsky, & S. Gershon (Eds.), *The behavior of psychiatric patients.* New York: Marcel Dekker.

Hanley, H. G., Stahl, S. M., & Freedman, D. X. (1977). Hyperserotonemia and amine metabolites in autistic and retarded children. *Archives of General Psychiatry, 34,* 521-531.

Hardesty, A. S. (1982). Behavioral assessment of children and adolescents. In E. I. Burdock, A. Sudilovsky, & S. Gershon (Eds.), *The behavior of psychiatric patients. Quantitative techniques for evaluation.* New York: Marcel Dekker.

Hassanyeh, F., & Davison, K. (1980). Bipolar affective psychosis with onset before age 16 years: Report of 10 cases. *British Journal of Psychiatry, 137,* 530-539.

Hayes, T. A., Logan Panitch, M., & Barker, E. (1975). Imipramine dosage in children: A comment on "imipramine and electrocardiographic abnormalities in hyperactive children." *American Journal of Psychiatry, 132,* 546-547.

Heninger, G. R. (1978). Lithium carbonate and brain function. I. Cerebral-evoked potentials, EEG, and symptom changes during lithium carbonate treatment. *Archives of General Psychiatry, 35*(2), 228-233.

Herjanic, B., & Campbell, W. (1977). Differentiating psychiatrically disturbed children on the basis of a structured interview. *Journal of Abnormal Child Psychology, 5,* 127-134.

Holliday, A. (1967). The problem of shifting definition of behavioral toxicity. In H. Brill, J. O. Cole, P. Deniker, H. Hippius, & P. B. Bradley (Eds.), *Neuropsychopharmacology.* Amsterdam: Excerpta Medica Foundation.

Holtzman, W. H. (1958). *The Holtzman ink blot technique.* New York: Psychological Corporation.

Horowitz, H. A. (1977). Lithium and the treatment of adolescent manic depressive illness. *Diseases of the Nervous System, 38,* 480-483.

Huessy, H. R., & Wright, A. L. (1970). The use of imipramine in children's behavior disorders. *Acta Paedopsychiatrica, 37,* 194-199.

ICD-9, International Classification of Diseases. (1977). *Manual of the International statistical classification of diseases, injuries, and causes of death* (Vol. 1). Geneva: World Health Organization.

Irwin, S. (1968). A rational framework for the development, evaluation, and use of psychoactive drugs. *American Journal of Psychiatry, 124*(Suppl.), 1-19.

Jefferson, J. W. (1982). The use of lithium in childhood and adolescence: An overview. *Journal of Clinical Psychiatry, 43*(5), 174-177.

Jefferson, J. W., Greist, J. H., & Ackerman, D. L. (1983). *Lithium Encyclopedia for Clinical Practice.* Madison, WI: Lithium Information Center.

Jefferson, J. W., Greist, J. H., & Baudhuin, M. (1981). Lithium: Interactions with other drugs. *Journal of Clinical Psychopharmacology, 1*(3), 124-134.

Jenner, F. A. (1979). Lithium and the question of kidney damage. *Archives of General Psychiatry, 36*(8 Spec. No.), 888-890.

Johnson, G., Maccario, M., Gershon, S., & Korein, J. (1970). The effects of lithium on electroencephalogram; behavior and serum electrolytes. *Journal of Nervous and Mental Disease, 151*(4), 273-289.

Judd, L. L. (1979). Effect of lithium on mood, cognition, and personality function in normal subjects. *Archives of General Psychiatry, 36*(7), 860-865.

Judd, L. L., Hubbard, B., Janowsky, D. S., Huey, L. Y., & Attewell, P. H. (1977). The effect of lithium carbonate on affect, mood and personality of normal subjects. *Archives of General Psychiatry, 34*(3), 346-351.

Judd, L. L., Hubbard, B., Janowsky, D. S., Huey, L. Y., & Takahashi, K. I. (1977). The effect of lithium carbonate on the cognitive functions of normal subjects. *Archives of General Psychiatry, 34*(3), 355-357.

Kajitani, T. (1963). Electroencephalographic studies of mentally retarded children. II. Effects of various psychotropic drugs on the electroencephalograms of mentally retarded children. *Psychiatria et Neurologia Japonica, 65*, 211-223.

Källén, B., & Tandberg, A. (1983). Lithium and pregnancy. *Acta Psychiatrica Scandinavica, 68*, 134-139.

Kane, J. J., & Smith, J. M. (1982). Tardive dyskinesia. Prevalence and risk factors, 1959 to 1979. *Archives of General Psychiatry, 39*, 473-481.

Kashani, J. H., Shekim, W. O., & Reid, J. C. (1984). Amitriptyline in children with major depressive disorder: A double-blind crossover pilot study. *Journal of the American Academy of Child Psychiatry, 23*, 348-351.

Kazamatsuri, H., Chien, C-p., Cole, J. O. (1973). Long-term treatment of tardive dyskinesia with haloperidol and tetrabenazine. *American Journal of Psychiatry, 130*(4), 479-483.

Kazdin, A. E. (1981). Assessment techniques for childhood depression: A critical appraisal. *Journal of the American Academy of Child Psychiatry, 20*, 358-375.

Kazdin, A. E., French, N. H., Unis, A. S., & Esveldt-Dawson, K. (1983). Assessment of childhood depression: Correspondence of child and parent ratings. *Journal of the American Academy of Child Psychiatry, 22*, 157-164.

Kazdin, A. E., & Petti, T. A. (1982). Self-report and interview measures of childhood and adolescent depression. *Journal of Child Psychology and Psychiatry, 23*, 437-457.

Kelly, J., Koch, M., & Buegel, D. (1976). Lithium carbonate in juvenile manic-depressive illness. *Diseases of the Nervous System, 37*, 90-92.

Kessler, K. A. (1978). Tricyclic antidepressants: Mode of action and clinical use. In M. A. Lipton, A. DiMascio, & K. F. Killam (Eds.), *Psychopharmacology: A generation of progress.* New York: Raven Press.

Klawans, H. L., Nausieda, P. A., Goetz, C. G., Tanner, C. M., & Weiner, W. J. (1982). Tourette-like symptoms following chronic neuroleptic therapy. In A. J. Friedhoff and T. N. Chase (Eds.), *Advances in Neurology, Vol. 35. Gilles de la Tourette Syndrome.* New York: Raven Press.

Klein, D. F., Gittelman, R., Quitkin, F., & Rifkin, A. (1980). *Diagnosis and drug treatment of psychiatric disorders: Adults and children* (2nd ed.). Baltimore: Williams & Wilkins.

Kline, A. H. (1968). Diazepam and the management of nocturnal enuresis. *Clinical Medicine, 75*, 20-22.

Kolko, D., Anderson, L. T., & Campbell, M. (1980). Sensory preference and overselective responding in autistic children. *Journal of Autism and Developmental Disorders, 10*, 259-271.

Kovács, M. (1980/81). Rating scales to assess depression in school-aged children. *Acta Paedopsychiatrica, 46*, 305-315.

Kraft, I. A., Ardali, C., Duffy, J. H., Hart, J. T., & Pearce, P. (1965). A clinical study of chlordiazepoxide used in psychiatric disorders of children. *International Journal of Neuropsychiatry, 1*, 433-437.

Krakowski, A. J. (1963). Chlordiazepoxide in treatment of children with emotional disturbances. *New York State Journal of Medicine, 63*, 3388-3392.

Kydd, R. R., & Werry, J. S. (1982). Schizophrenia in children under 16 years. *Journal of Autism and Developmental Disorders, 12*, 343-357.

Lader, M. H. (1984). Antianxiety drugs. In T. B. Karasu [Chair, American Psychiatric Commission on Psychiatric Therapies] *The Psychiatric Therapies*. Washington, DC: American Psychiatric Association.

Laska, E., Meisner, M., & Kushner, H. B. (1983). Optimal crossover designs in the presence of carryover effects. *Biometrics, 39*, 1087-1091.

La Veck, G. D., & Buckley, P. (1961). The use of psychopharmacologic agents in retarded children with behavior disorders. *Journal of Chronic Diseases, 13*, 174-183.

Law, W., III, Petti, T. A., & Kazdin, A. E. (1981). Withdrawal symptoms after graduated cessation of imipramine in children. *American Journal of Psychiatry, 138*, 647-650.

Lena, B. (1979). Lithium in child and adolescent psychiatry. *Archives of General Psychiatry, 36*, 854-855.

Lena, B., Surtees, S. J., & Maggs, R. (1978). The efficacy of lithium in the treatment of emotional disturbance in children and adolescents. In F. N. Johnson & S. Johnson (Eds.), *Lithium in medical practice*. Baltimore: University Park Press.

Linnoila, M., Saario, I., Maki, M. (1974). Effect of treatment with diazepam or lithium and alcohol on psychomotor skills related to driving. *European Journal of Clinical Pharmacology, 7*(5), 337-342.

Lipman, R. S., DiMascio, A., Reatig, N., & Kirson, T. (1978). Psychotropic drugs and mentally retarded children. In M. A. Lipton, A. DiMascio & K. F. Killam (Eds.), *Psychopharmacology: A generation of progress*. New York: Raven Press.

Lockyer, L., & Rutter, M. (1969). A five to fifteen year follow-up study of infantile psychosis. *British Journal of Psychiatry, 115*, 865-882.

Lorr, M., Jenkins, R. L., & Holsopple, J. Q. (1953). *Multidimensional scale for rating psychiatric patients, hospital form*. Technical Bulletin TB 10-507. Washington, DC: Veterans Administration.

Lowe, T. L., Cohen, D. J., Detlor, J., Kremenitzer, M. W., & Shaywitz, B. A. (1982). Stimulant medications precipitate Tourette's syndrome. *Journal of the American Medical Association, 247*(12), 1729-1731.

Lucas, A. R., & Pasley, F. C. (1969). Psychoactive drugs in the treatment of emotionally disturbed children: Haloperidol and diazepam. *Comprehensive Psychiatry, 10*(5), 376-386.

Lydiard, R. B., & Gelenberg, A. J. (1982). Hazards and adverse effects of lithium. *Annual Review of Medicine, 33,* 327-344.

MacLeod, C. M., Dekaban, A. S., & Hunt, E. (1978). Memory impairment in epileptic patients: Selective effects of phenobarbital concentration. *Science, 202,* 1102-1104.

Martini, L., & Ganong, W. F. (Eds.). (1971). *Frontiers in neuroendocrinology, 1971.* New York: Oxford University Press.

Mattes, J., & Gittelman, R. (1983). Growth of hyperactive children on maintenance methylphenidate. *Archives of General Psychiatry, 40,* 317-321.

McAndrew, J. B., Case, Q., & Treffert, D. A. (1972). Effects of prolonged phenothiazine intake on psychotic and other hospitalized children. *Journal of Autism and Childhood Schizophrenia, 2,* 75-91.

McConaghy, N. (1969). A controlled trial of imipramine, amphetamine, pad-and-bell conditioning and random awakening in the treatment of nocturnal enuresis. *Medical Journal of Australia, 2,* 237-239.

McGlashan, T. H., & Cleary, P. (1976). Clinical laboratory test standards for schizophrenic research subjects. *ECDEU Assessment Manual,* Publication No. (ADM) 76-338, 379-382. Washington, DC: Department of Health, Education & Welfare.

McGlashan, T. H., & Cleary, P. (1975). Clinical laboratory test standards for a sample of schizophrenics. *Psychopharmacologia, 44*(3), 281-285.

McKnew, D. H., Cytryn, L., Buchsbaum, M. S., Hamovit, J., Lamour, M., Rapoport, J. L., & Gershon, E. S. (1981). Lithium in children of lithium-responding parents. *Psychiatry Research, 4,* 171-180.

McNair, D. M. (1973). Antianxiety drugs and human performance. *Archives of General Psychiatry, 29*(11), 611-617.

McNutt, B. A., Boileau, R. A., Cohen, M. N., Sprague, R. L., & von Neumann, A. (1976). *The effects of long term stimulant medication on the growth and body composition of hyperactive children: II Report on 2 years.* Paper presented at the Annual Early Clinical Drug Evaluation Unit Meeting, Psychopharmacology Research Branch, National Institute of Mental Health, Key Biscayne.

Meiselas, K., Peselow, E. D., Die Trill, M. L., Deutsch, S. I., Perry, R., Cicero, S. D., & Campbell, M. (1984). *Neuroleptic-related dyskinesias in children with a high baseline rate of abnormal movements: Methodological issues.* Paper presented at the 31st Annual Meeting of the American Academy of Science Psychiatry, Toronto.

Messerschmitt, P. L. (1972). *L'utilization du pimozide en pédo-psychiatrie (à propos de 186 malades).* Faculté de Médicine de Paris: Theses.

Mikkelsen, E. J., Detlor, J., & Cohen, D. J. (1981). School avoidance and social phobia triggered by haloperidol in patients with Tourette's disorder. *American Journal of Psychiatry, 138*(12), 1572-1576.

Mikkelsen, E. J., Rapoport, J. L., Nee, L., Gruenau, C., Mendelson, W., & Gillin, J. C. (1980). Childhood enuresis. I. Sleep patterns and psychopathology. *Archives of General Psychiatry, 37,* 1139-1144.

Murburg, M., Anton, R. F., Nelson, J. C., & Jatlow, P. I. (1982). Noninvasive measurement of cardiac ejection fraction during desipramine treatment. *Psychosomatics, 23*(7), 759-761.

Naruse, H., Nagahata, M., Nakane, Y., Shirahashi, K., Takesada, M., & Yamazaki, K. (1982). A multicenter double-blind trial of pimozide [Orap], haloperidol and placebo in children with behavioral disorders, using crossover design. *Acta Paedopsychiatrica, 48,* 173-184.

Overall, J. E., & Gorham, D. R. (1962). The brief psychiatric rating scale. *Psychological Report, 10,* 799-812.

Pangalia-Ratulangi, E. A. (1973). Pilot evaluation of Orap® (Pimozide, R6238). *Child Psychiatry, Psychiatria, Neurologia, Neurochirugia, 76,* 17-27.

Paulson, G. W., Rizvi, C. A., & Crane, G. E. (1975). Tardive dyskinesia as a possible sequel of long-term therapy with phenothiazines. *Clinical Pediatrics, 14,* 953-955.

Perry, R., Campbell, M., Green, W. H., Small, A. M., Die Trill, M. L., Meiselas, K., Golden, R. R., & Deutsch, S. I. (1985). Neuroleptic-related dyskinesias in autistic children: A prospective study. *Psychopharmacology Bulletin, 21*(1), 140-143.

Perry, R., Campbell, M., Grega, D. M., & Anderson, L. (1984). Saliva lithium levels in children: Their use in monitoring serum lithium levels and lithium side effects. *Journal of Clinical Psychopharmacology, 4,* 199-202.

Pesikoff, R. B., & Davis, P. C. (1971). Treatment of pavor nocturnus and somnambulism in children. *American Journal of Psychiatry, 128,* 778-781.

Petti, T. A. (1978). Depression in hospitalized child psychiatry patients: Approaches to measuring depression. *Journal of the American Academy of Child Psychiatry, 17,* 49-59.

Petti, T. A. (in press). Psychopharmacologic treatment of anxiety disorders in children and adolescents. In J. F. McDermott (Eds.), *Panel on Treatment of Anxiety Disorders of Childhood and Adolescents.* (In T. B. Karasu [Chair] Psychiatric Treatment Manual 1). Washington, DC: American Psychiatric Association.

Petti, T. A., & Campbell, M. (1975). Imipramine and seizures. *American Journal of Psychiatry, 132,* 538-540.

Petti, T. A., Fish, B., Shapiro, T., Cohen, I. L., & Campbell, M. (1982). Effects of chlordiazepoxide in disturbed children: a pilot study. *Journal of Clinical Psychopharmacology, 2*(4), 270-273.

Petti, T. A., & Law, W., III (1981). Abrupt cessation of high-dose imipramine treatment in children. *Journal of the American Medical Association, 246,* 768-769.

Petti, T. A., & Law, W., III (1982). Imipramine treatment of depressed children: A double-blind pilot study. *Journal of Clinical Psychopharmacology, 2,* 107-110.

Pharmacotherapy of Children [special issue]. (1973). *Psychopharmacology Bulletin.*

Physician's Desk Reference. (1985). Oradell, NJ: Medical Economics Co.

Pilkington, T. L. (1961). Comparative effects of librium and taractan on behavior disorders of mentally retarded children. *Diseases of the Nervous System, 22,* 573-575.

Platt, J. E., Campbell, M., Green, W. H., & Grega, D. M. (1984). Cognitive effects of lithium carbonate and haloperidol in treatment-resistant aggressive children. *Archives of General Psychiatry, 41,* 657-662.

Polizos, P., & Engelhardt, D. M. (1980). Dyskinetic and neurological complications in children treated with psychotropic medication. In W. E. Fann, R. C. Smith, J. M. Davis, & E. F. Domino (Eds.), *Tardive dyskinesia. Research and treatment.* Jamaica, New York: Spectrum Publications.

Polizos, P., Engelhardt, D. M., Hoffman, S. P., & Waizer, J. (1973). Neurological consequences of psychotropic drug withdrawal in schizophrenic children. *Journal of Autism and Childhood Schizophrenia, 3,* 247-253.

Pool, D., Bloom, W., Mielke. D. H., Roniger, J. J., & Gallant, D. M. (1976). A controlled evaluation of loxitane in seventy-five adolescent schizophrenic patients. *Current Therapeutic Research, 19,* 99-104.

Poussaint, A. F., & Ditman, K. S. (1965). A controlled study of imipramine (tofranil) in the treatment of childhood enuresis. *Journal of Pediatrics, 67,* 283-290.

Poznanski, E. O., Cook, S. C., & Carroll, B. J. (1979). A depression rating scale for children. *Pediatrics, 64,* 442-450.

Prange, A. J., Jr. (Ed.). (1974). *The thyroid axis, drugs, and behavior.* New York: Raven Press.

Pregelj, S., & Barkauskas, A. (1967). Thioridazine in the treatment of mentally retarded children. A four-year retroactive evaluation. *Journal of the Canadian Psychiatric Association, 12,* 213-215.

Preskorn, S. H., Weller, E. B., & Weller, R. A. (1982). Depression in children: Relationship between plasma imipramine levels and response. *Journal of Clinical Psychiatry, 43,* 450-453.

Preskorn, S. H., Weller, E. B., Weller, R. A., & Glotzbach, E. (1983). Plasma levels of imipramine and adverse effects in children. *American Journal of Psychiatry, 140,* 1332-1335.

Prien, R. J. (1979). Lithium in the prophylactic treatment of affective disorders. *Archives of General Psychiatry, 36,* 847-848.

Psychopharmacology Bulletin. (1973). Special issue on pharmacotherapy of children.

Puig-Antich, J. (1980). Affective disorders in childhood: a review and perspective. *Psychiatric Clinics of North America, 3*(3), 403-424.

Puig-Antich, J. (1984). *Depression in children and adolescents.* Paper presented at the New York Council on Child Psychiatry, New York.

Puig-Antich, J., Blau, S., Marx, N., Greenhill, L. L., & Chambers, W. (1978). Prepubertal major depressive disorder. A pilot study. *Journal of the American Academy of Child Psychiatry, 17,* 695-707.

Puig-Antich, J. Greenhill, L. L., Sassin, J., & Sachar, E. J. (1978). Growth hormone, prolactin and cortisol responses and growth patterns in hyperkinetic children treated with dextro-amphetamine. *Journal of the American Academy of Child Psychiatry, 17,* 457-475.

Puig-Antich, J., Perel, J. M., Lupatkin, W., Chambers, W. J., Shea, C., Tabrizi, M. A., & Stiller, R. L. (1979). Plasma levels of imipramine (IMI) and desmethylimipramine (DMI) and clinical response in prepubertal major depressive disorder, a preliminary report. *Journal of the American Academy of Child Psychiatry, 18,* 616-627.

Puig-Antich, J., Perel, J., Lupatkin, W., Chambers, W. J., Tabrizi, M. A., Goetz, J., Davies, M., & Stiller, R. (in press). Imipramine in prepubertal major depressive disorders. *Archives of General Psychiatry.*

Quinn, P. O., & Rapoport, J. L. (1975). One-year follow-up of hyperactive boys treated with imipramine or methylphenidate. *American Journal of Psychiatry, 132*(3), 241-245.

Rainey, J. M. (1982). *Q-T prolongation in schizophrenia.* Paper presented at the Annual Meeting of the Society of Biological Psychiatry, Toronto.

Rapoport, J. (1965). Childhood behavior and learning problems treated with imipramine. *International Journal of Neuropsychiatry, 1,* 635-642.

Rapoport, J. L., Abramson, A., Alexander, D., & Lott, I. (1971). Playroom observations of hyperactive children on medication. *Journal of the American Academy of Child Psychiatry, 10,* 524-534.

Rapoport, J. L., Buchsbaum, M. S., Weingartner, H., Zahn, T. P., Ludlow, C., & Mikkelsen, E. J. (1980). Dextroamphetamine: Its cognitive and behavioral effects in normal and hyperactive boys and normal men. *Archives of General Psychiatry, 37,* 933-943.

Rapoport, J. L., Buchsbaum, M. S., Zahn, T. P., Weingartner, H., Ludlow, C., & Mikkelsen, E. J. (1978a). Dextroamphetamine: Cognitive and behavioral effects in normal prepubertal boys. *Science, 199,* 560-563.

Rapoport, J. L., & Ismond, D. R. (1984). *DSM-III training guide for diagnosis of childhood disorders.* New York: Brunner/Mazel.

Rapoport, J. L., Mikkelsen, E. J., & Werry, J. S. (1978). Antimanic, antianxiety, hallucinogenic and miscellaneous drugs. In J. S. Werry (Ed.), *Pediatric psychopharmacology: The use of behavioral modifying drugs in children.* New York: Brunner/Mazel.

Rapoport, J. L., Mikkelsen, E. J., Zavadil, A., Nee, L., Gruenau, C., Mendelson, W., & Gillin, J. C. (1980). Childhood enuresis, II. Psychopathology, tricyclic concentration in plasma, and antienuretic effects. *Archives of General Psychiatry, 37,* 1146-1152.

Rapoport, J. L., Quinn, P. O., Bradbard, G., Riddle, K. D., & Brooks, E. (1974). Imipramine and methylphenidate treatments of hyperactive boys. A double-blind comparison. *Archives of General Psychiatry, 30,* 789-793.

Realmuto, G. M., Erickson, W. D., Yellin, A. M., Hopwood, J. H., & Greenberg, L. M. (1984). Clinical comparison of thiothixene and thioridazine in schizophrenic adolescents. *American Journal of Psychiatry, 141*(3), 440-442.

Reisberg, B., & Gershon, S. (1979). Side effects associated with lithium therapy. *Archives of General Psychiatry, 36,* 879-887.

Rifkin, A., Quitkin, F., Carrillo, C., Blumberg, A. G., & Klein, D. F. (1972). Lithium carbonate in emotionally unstable character disorder. *Archives of General Psychiatry, 27,* 519-523.

Ritvo, E. R., Freeman, B. J., Geller, E., & Yuwiler, A. (1983). Effects of fenfluramine on 14 outpatients with the syndrome of autism. *Journal of the American Academy of Child Psychiatry, 22,* 549-558.

Ritvo, E. R., Freeman, B. J., Yuwiler, A., Geller, E., Yokota, Y., Schroth, P., & Novak, P. (1984). Study of fenfluramine in outpatients with the syndrome of autism. *Journal of Pediatrics, 105*(5), 823-828.

Ritvo, E., Yuwiler, A., Geller, E., Ornitz, E. M., Saeger, K., & Plotkin, S. (1970). Increased blood serotonin and platelets in early infantile autism. *Archives of General Psychiatry, 23,* 566-572.

Rivera-Calimlim, L., Nasrallah, H., Strauss, J., & Lasagna, L. (1976). Clinical response and plasma levels: Effect of dose, dosage schedules, and drug interactions on plasma chlorpromazine levels. *American Journal of Psychiatry, 133,* 646-652.

Robins, L. N. (1966). *Deviant children grown up.* Baltimore: William & Wilkins.

Roche, A. F., Lipman, R. A., Overall, J. E., & Hung, W. E. (1979). The effects of stimulant medication on the growth of hyperkinetic children. *Pediatrics, 63,* 847-850.

Ross, M. S., & Moldofsky, H. (1977). Comparison of pimozide with haloperidol in Gilles de la Tourette's syndrome. *Lancet, 1,* 103.

Sachar, E. J. (Ed.). (1976). *Hormones, behavior, and psychopathology.* New York: Raven Press.

Safer, D., Allen, R., & Barr, E. (1972). Depression of growth in hyperactive children on stimulant drugs. *New England Journal of Medicine, 287*(5), 217-220.

Saraf, K. R., Klein, D. F., Gittelman-Klein, R., Gootman, N., & Greenhill, P. (1978). EKG effects of imipramine treatment in children. *Journal of the American Academy of Child Psychiatry, 17,* 60-69.

Satterfield, J. H., Cantwell, D. P., Schell, A., & Blaschke, T. (1979). Growth of hyperactive children treated with methylphenidate. *Archives of General Psychiatry, 36,* 212-217.

Schooler, N. R., & Kane, J. M. (1982). Research diagnoses for tardive dyskinesia. *Archives of General Psychiatry, 39*(4), 486-487.

Schou, M. (1968). Lithium in psychiatric therapy and prophylaxis. *Journal of Psychiatric Research 6*(1), 67-95.

Schou, M. (1969). Lithium: Elimination rate, dosage, control, poisoning, goiter, mode of action. *Acta Psychiatrica Scandinavica, 207* (Suppl.), 49-59.

Schou, M. (1979). Lithium as a prophylactic agent in unipolar affective illness. *Archives of General Psychiatry, 36,* 849-851.

Schou, M. (1981). *Lithium: Psychopharmacology update. Chronic treatment, drug interactions and side effects.* Paper presented at the Seventh Annual International Symposium on Psychopharmacology, Louisville.

Schou, M. (1983). Lithium and relapse prevention in manic-depressive illness. *Psychosomatics, 24,* 533-541.

Schou, M., & Vestergaard, P. (1981). Lithium and the kidney scare. [Editorial]. *Psychosomatics, 22,* 92-94.

Schulterbrandt, J. G., & Raskin, A. (1977). Depression in childhood: Diagnosis, treatment, and conceptual models. Raven Press: New York.

Shader, R. I., & DiMascio, A. (1970). *Psychotropic drug side effects.* Baltimore: Williams & Wilkins.

Shagas, C., & Straumanis, J. J. (1978). Drugs and human sensory evoked potentials. In M. A. Lipton, A. DiMascio, & K. F. Killam (Eds.), *Psychopharmacology: A generation of progress.* New York: Raven Press.

Shapiro, A. K., & Shapiro, E. (1981). Do stimulants provoke, cause or exacerbate tics and Tourette's syndrome? *Comprehensive Psychiatry, 22*(3), 265-273.

Shapiro, A. K., & Shapiro, E. (1982). Clinical efficacy of haloperidol, pimozide, penfluridol, and clonidine in the treatment of Tourette syndrome. In A. J. Friendhoff & T. N. Chase (Eds.), *Advances in Neurology, Vol. 35. Gilles de la Tourette syndrome.* New York: Raven Press.

Shapiro, A. K., & Shapiro, E. (1984). Controlled study of pimozide vs. placebo in Tourette's syndrome. *Journal of the American Academy of Child Psychiatry, 23,* 161-173.

Shaywitz, S. E., Hunt, R. D., Jatlow, P., Cohen, D. J., Young, J. G., Pierce, R. N., Anderson, G. M., & Shaywitz, B. A. (1982). Psychopharmacology of attention deficit disorder: Pharmacokinetic, neuroendocrine, and behavioral measures following acute and chronic treatment with methylphenidate. *Pediatrics, 69,* 688-694.

Sheard, M. H. (1975). Lithium in the treatment of aggression. *Journal of Nervous and Mental Disease, 160*(1), 108-118.

Sheard, M. H., Marini, J. L., Bridges, C. I., & Wagner, E. (1976). The effect of lithium on impulsive, aggressive behavior in man. *American Journal of Psychiatry, 133*(12), 1409-1413.

Shopsin, B., & Gershon, S. (1973). Pharmacology-toxicology of the lithium ion. In S. Gershon & B. Shopsin (Eds.), *Lithium: Its role in psychiatric research and treatment.* New York: Plenum Press.

Shopsin, B., Gershon, S., & Pinckney, L. (1969). The secretion of lithium in human mixed saliva: Effects of ingested lithium on electrolyte distribution in saliva and serum. *International Pharmacopsychiatry, 2,* 148-169.

Shopsin, B., Gershon, S., Thompson, H., & Collins, P. (1975). Psychoactive drugs in mania: A controlled comparison of lithium carbonate, chlorpromazine, and haloperidol. *Archives of General Psychiatry, 32,* 34-42.

Siassi, I. (1982). Lithium treatment of impulsive behavior in children. *Journal of Clinical Psychiatry, 43*(12), 482-484.

Simeon, J., Saletu, B., Saletu, M., Itil, T. M., DaSilva, J. (1973). *Thiothixene in childhood psychoses.* Paper presented at the Third International Symposium on phenothiazines, Rockville, Maryland.

Simon, G. B., & Gilles, S. M. (1964). Some physical characteristics of a group of psychotic children. *British Journal of Psychiatry, 110,* 104-107.

Simpson, G. M. (1982). Neurological assessments. In E. I. Burdock, A. Sudilovsky, & S. Gershon (Eds.), *The behavior of psychiatric patients.* New York: Marcel Dekker.

Simpson, G. M., Amuso, D., Blair, J. H., & Farkas, T. (1964). Aspects of phenothiazine-produced extrapyramidal symptoms. *Archives of General Psychiatry, 10*(2), 199-208.

Simpson, G. M., & Angus, J.W.S. (1970). A rating scale for extrapyramidal side effects. *Acta Psychiatrica Scandinavica,* (Suppl. 212), 11-19.

Simpson, G. M., Lee, J. H., Zoubok, B., & Gardos, G. (1979). A rating scale for tardive dyskinesia. *Psychopharmacology (Berlin), 64*(2), 171-179.

Singh, N. N., & Aman, M. G. (1981). Effects of thioridazine dosage on the behavior of severely mentally retarded persons. *American Journal of Mental Deficiency, 85,* 580-587.

Sleator, E. K., von Neumann, A., & Sprague, R. L. (1974). Hyperactive children: A continuous long-term placebo-controlled follow-up. *Journal of the American Medical Association, 229*(3), 316-317.

Small, J. G., Milstein, V., Perez, H. C., Small, I. F., & Moore, F. (1972). EEG and neurophysiological studies of lithium in normal volunteers. *Biological Pharmacy, 5,* 65-77.

Smith, R. C., Tamminga, C. A., Haraszti, J., Pandey, G. N., & Davis, J. M. (1977). Effects of dopamine agonists in tardive dyskinesia. *American Journal of Psychiatry, 134*(7), 763-768.

Spitzer, R. L., Endicott, J., & Robins, E. (1978). Research diagnostic criteria. *Archives of General Psychiatry, 35,* 773-782.

Sprague, R. L. (1973). Recommended performance measures for psychotropic drug investigations. *Psychopharmacology Bulletin* [Special Issue, Pharmacotherapy of Children], 85-88.

Sprague, R. L. (1978). Principles of clinical trials, and social, ethical and legal issues of drug use in children. In J. S. Werry (Ed.), *Pediatric psychopharmacology: The use of behavior modifying drugs in children.* New York: Brunner/Mazel.

Sprague, R. L., & Sleator, E. K. (1977). Methylphenidate in hyperkinetic children: Differences in dose effects on learning and social behavior. *Science, 198,* 1274-1276.

Sprague, R. L., & Werry, J. S. (1971). Methodology of psychopharmacological studies with the retarded. In N. R. Ellis (Ed.), *International review of research in mental retardation.* New York: Academic Press.

Sprague, R. L., & Werry, J. S. (1973). Pediatric psychopharmacology. *Psychopharmacology Bulletin* [Special Issue, Pharmacotherapy of Children], 21-23.

Spring, G., & Frankel, M. (1981). New data on lithium and haloperidol incompatibility. *American Journal of Psychiatry, 138,* 818-821.

Stahl, S. M. (1980). Tardive Tourette syndrome in an autistic patient after long-term neuroleptic administration. *American Journal of Psychiatry, 137,* 1267-1269.

Stores, G. (1978). Antiepileptics (anticonvulsants). In J. S. Werry (Ed.), *Pediatric psychopharmacology. The use of behavior modifying drugs in children.* New York: Brunner/Mazel.

Tanner, J. M. (1973). Physical growth and development. In J. O. Forfar & G. C. Arneil (Eds.), *Textbook of paediatrics.* Edinburgh: Churchill Livingstone.

Tanner, J. M., Whitehouse, R. H., Hughes, P.C.R., & Vince, F. P. (1971). Effect of human growth hormone treatment for 1 to 7 years on growth of 100 children, with growth hormone deficiency, low birthweight, inherited smallness, Turner's Syndrome and other complaints. *Archives of Disease in Childhood, 46,* 745-782.

Tarjan, C., Lowery, V. E., & Wright, S. W. (1957). Use of chlorpromazine in 278 mentally deficient patients. *American Medical Association Journal of Disturbed Children, 94,* 294-300.

Thompson, T., & Schuster, C. R. (1968). *Behavioral pharmacology.* Englewood Cliffs, NJ: Prentice-Hall.

Valentine, A. A., & Maxwell, C. (1968). Enuresis in severely subnormal children—a clinical trial of imipramine. *Journal of Mental Subnormality, 14,* 84-90.

van der Kolk, B. A., Shader, R. I., & Greenblatt, D. J. (1978). Autonomic effects of psychotropic drugs. In M. A. Lipton, A. DiMascio, & K. F. Killam (Eds.), *Psychopharmacology: A generation of progress.* New York: Raven Press.

Van Der Velde, C. D. (1970). Effectiveness of lithium carbonate in the treatment of manic depressive illness. *American Journal of Psychiatry, 127*(3), 345-351.

Van Putten, T., May, P.R.A., & Marder, S. R. (1984). Akathisia with haloperidol and thiothixene. *Archives of General Psychiatry, 41,* 1036-1039.

Varley, C. K., & Trupin, E. W. (1982). Double-blind administration of methylphenidate to mentally retarded children with attention deficit disorder: A preliminary study. *American Journal of Mental Deficiency, 86,* 560-566.

Villenueve, A. (1972). The rabbit syndrome. A peculiar extrapyramidal reaction. *Canadian Psychiatric Association Journal, 17,* 69-72.

Waizer, J., Hoffman, S. P., Polizos, P., & Engelhardt, D. M. (1974). Outpatient treatment of hyperactive school children with imipramine. *American Journal of Psychiatry, 131,* 587-591.

Waizer, J., Polizos, P., Hoffman, S. P., Engelhardt, D. M., & Margolis, R. A. (1972). A single-blind evaluation of thiothixene with outpatient schizophrenic children. *Journal of Autism and Childhood Schizophrenia, 2,* 378-386.

Walker, M. (1982). The psychomotor stimulants. In S. E. Bruening & A. D. Poling (Eds.), *Drugs and Mental Retardation.* Springfield, IL: Charles C Thomas.

Warneke, L. (1975). A case of manic-depressive illness in childhood. *Canadian Psychiatric Association Journal, 20,* 195-200.

Weinberg, W. A., Rutman, J., Sullivan, L., Penick, E. C., & Dietz, S. G. (1973). Depression in children referred to an educational diagnostic center: Diagnosis and treatment—preliminary report. *Journal of Pediatrics, 83,* 1065-1072.

Weiss, G., Hechtman, L., Perlman, T., Hopkins, J., & Wener, A. (1979). Hyperactives as young adults: A controlled prospective ten-year follow-up of 75 children. *Archives of General Psychiatry, 36,* 675-681.

Weller, E. B., Preskorn, S. H., Weller, R. A., & Croskell, M. (1983). Childhood depression: Imipramine levels and response. *Psychopharmacology Bulletin, 19*(1), 59-62.

Weller, E. B., Weller, R. A., Preskorn, S. H., & Glotzbach, R. (1982). Steady-state plasma imipramine levels in prepubertal depressed children. *American Journal of Psychiatry, 139,* 506-508.

Wender, P. H. (1971). *Minimal brain dysfunction in children.* New York: Wiley-Interscience.

Werry, J. S. (1978). Measures in pediatric psychopharmacology. In J. S. Werry (Ed.), *Pediatric psychopharmacology: The use of behavior modifying drugs in children.* New York: Brunner/Mazel.

Werry, J. S. (1979). Behavior observations and activity measures for use in pediatric psychopharmacology. Pp. 80-100 in *Guidelines for the Clinical Evaluation of Psychoactive Drugs in Infants and Children.* Stock no. 017-012-00281-1, U.S. Department of Health, Education, and Welfare, Public Health Service, Food and Drug Administration. Washington, DC: Government Printing Office.

Werry, J. S., & Aman, M. G. (1975). Methylphenidate and haloperidol in children. *Archives of General Psychiatry, 32*(6), 790-795.

Werry, J. S., Aman, M. G., & Diamond, E. (1980). Imipramine and methylphenidate in hyperactive children. *Journal of Child Psychology and Psychiatry, 21,* 27-35.

Werry, J. S., Aman, M. G., & Lampen, E. (1975). Haloperidol and methylphenidate in hyperactive children. *Acta Paedopsychiatrica, 42,* 26-40.

Werry, J. S., Weiss, G., Douglas, V., & Martin, J. (1966). Studies on the hyperactive child: III. The effect of chlorpromazine upon behavior and learning ability. *Journal of the American Academy of Child Psychiatry, 5,* 292-312.

White, J. W., & O'Shanick, G. (1977). Juvenile manic-depressive illness. *American Journal of Psychiatry, 134*(9), 1035-1036.

Whitehead, P. L., & Clark, L. D. (1970). Effect of lithium carbonate, placebo, and thioridazine on hyperactive children. *American Journal of Psychiatry, 127*(6), 824-825.

Winsberg, B. G., Bialer, I., Kupietz, S., & Tobias, J. (1972). Effects of imipramine and dextroamphetamine on behavior of neuropsychiatrically impaired children. *American Journal of Psychiatry, 128,* 109-115.

Winsberg, B. G., Goldstein, S., Yepes, L. E., & Perel, J. M. (1975). Imipramine and electrocardiographic abnormalities in hyperactive children. *American Journal of Psychiatry, 132,* 542-545.

Winsberg, B. G., Kupietz, S. S., Sverd, J., Hungund, B. L., & Young, N. L. (1982). Methylphenidate oral dose plasma concentrations and behavioral response in children. *Psychopharmacology, 76,* 329-332.

Wittenborn, J. R. (1978). Behavioral toxicity in normal humans as a model for assessing behavioral toxicity in patients. In M. A. Lipton, A. DiMascio, & K. F. Killam (Eds.), *Psychopharmacology: A generation of progress.* New York: Raven Press.

Wolpert, A., Hagamen, M. B., & Merlis, S. (1967). A comparative study of thiothixene and trifluoperazine in childhood schizophrenia. *Current Therapeutic Research, 9,* 482-485.

Wong, G. H., & Cock, R. J. (1971). Long-term effects of haloperidol on severely emotionally disturbed children. *Australian and New Zealand Journal of Psychiatry, 5,* 296-300.

Youngerman, J., & Canino, I. A. (1978). Lithium carbonate use in children and adolescents. *Archives of General Psychiatry, 35,* 216-224.

Youngerman, J. K., & Canino, I. A. (1983). Violent kids, violent parents: Family pharmacotherapy. *American Journal of Orthopsychiatry, 53*(1), 152-156.

Zrull, J. P., Westman, J. C., Arthur, B., & Bell, W. A. (1963). A comparison of chlordiazepoxide, d-amphetamine, and placebo in the treatment of the hyperkinetic syndrome in children. *American Journal of Psychiatry, 120,* 590-591.

Zrull, J. P., Westman, J. C., Arthur, B., & Rice, D. L. (1964). Comparison of diazepam, d-amphetamine and placebo in the treatment of the hyperkinetic syndrome in children. *American Journal of Psychiatry, 121,* 388-389.

INDEX

ABOUT THE AUTHORS

Magda Campbell, M. D., is Professor of Psychiatry and Director of the Children's Psychopharmacology Unit at the New York University Medical Center. She has been the recipient of several National Institute of Mental Health research grants in the field of psychopharmacology in children. Dr. Campbell has served on many state and federal advisory committees and task forces that oversee pharmacological treatment of disturbed children. She has published extensively, is a well-known speaker, and is internationally recognized as a senior researcher in the field.

Wayne H. Green, M. D., and Stephen I. Deutsch, M.D., Ph.D., are members of the interdisciplinary research team with Dr. Campbell. Both have published extensively in the field of childhood disorders, with particular reference to psychopharmacology.

Although the above group represents a collaborative team that has made important research and clinical contributions, each is individually recognized for his or her research.